Achieving
Natural Quiet

Dr Earl Mindell

IMPORTANT

This book is intended not as a substitute for personal medical advice but as a supplement to that advice for the patient who wishes to understand more about their condition.

Before taking any form of treatment YOU SHOULD ALWAYS CONSULT YOUR MEDICAL PRACTITIONER .

FIRST PUBLISHED BY HILITE PUBLISHING - 2013
ASH HOUSE, ASH ROAD, LONGFIELD, KENT DA3 8SA

© Dr Earl Mindell

ISBN 978-1-899205-18-9

Printed and bound in Great Britain

About the author, Dr. Earl Mindell - *best-selling author and world's foremost authority on nutritional supplements.*

Generally recognized as the Father of the Nutritional Revolution, Dr. Earl Mindell literally wrote the book on dietary supplements. His Vitamin Bible has sold 11 million copies and has been translated into 30 languages, making it the best-selling nutritional book of all time.

As a Doctor of Nutrition, certified pharmacist and Master Herbalist, Dr. Mindell is the number one authority on both nutritional supplements and traditional drugs. He has often been called America's Most Trusted Pharmacist.

Altogether, Dr. Mindell has authored more than 50 books, on health, nutrition and pharmacology, along with scores of articles and professional papers.

He has also been interviewed on hundreds of radio and TV programmes around the world including CNN, Live with Regis, Good Morning America, The Oprah Winfrey Show, The David Letterman Show and Canada AM. He has also been positively profiled in USA Today and The Wall Street Journal among many other publications.

Frequently invited to speak at health conferences and seminars throughout the world, Dr. Mindell has shared the stage with former U.S. Presidents Gerald Ford and George H.W. Bush, former U.S. Senator Bob Dole, former U.S. Secretary of State Colin Powell, former New York City Mayor Rudy Giuliani, former British Prime Minister Margaret Thatcher, Business Leader Steven Forbes, and Actor Christopher Reeve, among many others.

As a result of his long-time contributions and dedication, Dr. Mindell received the prestigious President's Award given by the National Nutritional Foods Association (NNFA) in 2002. He was also inducted into the California Pharmacy Hall of Fame in February 2007. He is a Fellow at the British Institute of Homeopathy, and also serves as a Director for the Corporate Board for the Illinois College of Physicians and Surgeons.

Table of Contents

1 Introduction

Throughout history, mankind has experienced the most crippling and ravaging sufferings. A number of factors have targeted humanity with morbid effects ranging from the sublime to the ridiculous, leaving every part of the populated world ravaged. These factors can be severe diseases or specified clinical conditions that can bring dramatic disturbances to one's life or even perish a precious life, from the face of the earth. Nevertheless, the power of positive thinking and constructive behaviour can create the most favourable situations even from the realms of most inevitable. Comprehensive knowledge and improved understanding of your illness can guide your thoughts and attitudes that will lead you to accomplish complete recovery.

A comprehensive account of psychological influences on a man's life can provide the basis of successful therapeutics for treating both psychological and medical illnesses. The history of this practice is very short, only limited to last a few decades. Unawareness about psychological conflicts affects the quality of life without coming into conscious notice. Almost every disease or disorder has its own physical and psychological repercussions; there are a few distinctive illnesses or diseases that possess both psychological and physiological symptoms and causes that are relatively more pronounced and tinnitus is thought to be among those very few.

Tinnitus is a medical and psychological condition and not

specifically a disease. Tinnitus, 'ringing in the ears' is a dominating and weakening disorder. It is presently affecting more than 15% of the world's population and in addition, tinnitus seriously disturbs the quality of life of around 3% of them. Incidentally, it is easier to talk about other disorders in which physiological factors lead to the development of psychological symptoms and vice versa. But in case of tinnitus it is rather difficult to find that exact relationship between physiological and psychological factors. As a result, it becomes even harder to find its relevant treatment and an obvious cure. It is imperative to understand and develop a clinical investigative approach, together with subjective observations, to diagnose causes and symptoms of tinnitus. All these and many more inconclusive trials and uncontrolled treatments have made it even harder and inevitable to solve the problem of tinnitus in the past. Throughout the last century limited knowledge and incompatible resources have resulted in difficulties in coming up with a proper treatment for this disorder.

In the last few years, major and precise methods have been developed to address this disorder. It can be now confirmed that a significant and comprehensive classification of causes and symptoms for tinnitus has been made to resolve these difficulties that have existed for decades. Latest scientific tools are emerging and thus tinnitus can be treated reliably by strong nutritional/supplemental approach *(i.e. Natural Quiet, see page 106),* electrical stimulant devices, specific tones, other types of sounds and medical prescriptions.

We should be able to clarify certain areas that are related to strategy and understanding of tinnitus. In particular, we need to discuss and find answers to some questions that clearly highlight the need of information on tinnitus. First of all, there are several causes of tinnitus and the main reasons for different forms of this particular disorder; so more scientific classification must be established with a therapeutic value. Secondly, what are the main reasons (either environmental or medical) that participate in causing ringing in the ears? What are the fundamental and implicit pathophysiological mechanisms? Whether different forms of tinnitus are related to each other? Can a person be affected by different forms at the same time? What the parameters should be of the severity of the condition? What kind of treatment should be followed for specific form of ringing in the ears? All these and many more questions should be answered to increase the rate of successful rehabilitation of impaired individuals.

A very crucial point to be considered is that, if the cause of the suffering is unknown, then all the follow-ups will mostly be just speculations. In this scenario the classification will be incomplete and incorrect. Whereas a treatment mislead to false, practice due to general acceptance of inappropriate guidelines. Noticeably, the previous classifications of tinnitus into objective and subjective forms have also caused difficulties in its treatment. The previous classification was not completely wrong but was just not good enough. It is evident that clear and prospective classification is of core value towards broad and thorough treatment of tinnitus in the future. Hence, the refusal to the importance of classification will result in complete chaos in the thoughts of patients who have been waiting for the right solution for their problem.

Nature has its resources to fluctuate and influence the frequency of living standards of Mankind. Sometimes it can be merely influential and sometimes can be really devastating. It can cause serious damage as well as can take many lives. Sound is one of Mother Nature's definite sensations that can be associated with harming qualities related to hearing mechanism. Sound can be produced externally as in the case of the new invention of electric stimulation of cochlea (auditory portion of internal ear). Some authenticated researches have proved that cochlea is itself capable of producing sound. These sounds are tiny, but recordable acoustic oscillations. However, this does not include classification of tinnitus until the patients claim to hear these oscillations.

Further classification of tinnitus can be made on the basis of generating source of the sound or noises. This classification enables clinicians and practitioners to evaluate the accurate condition of the patient. The emergence of these sites is mostly observed; middle ear, outer ear, sensory organ of hearing, auditory nerve and brain stem. Wax in the ear canal can also cause tinnitus, and tinnitus can also lead to other ear diseases and malfunctioning of the ears such as deafness. Unfortunately, complete recovery of such diseases does not mean that tinnitus will go away as well. This can be due to the fact that the origin of tinnitus can be different from lesion of that specific disease.

Tinnitus is a sensation that can last from seconds to several minutes and then gradually the time frame expands and minutes turn into hours. The episodes can be spontaneous, prolonged and periodic and these sensations can be caused due to certain noise exposure. This exposure can also result in slight injury to the ear. High frequency sound, like music through a heavy sound system or noise of a cracker, can initiate ringing in the ears. Such ringing can be heard in one ear at a time or in both the ears at the same time. Tinnitus disorder can occur in anybody at any stage of their life. It may prevail in a child, adolescent, young, old, males and females regardless of age, gender or habitat. Nevertheless, the prevalence rate is higher in men, factory workers, patients with hypertension and arteriosclerosis. One thing that can be common among all patients is that the more they have hearing problems the more likely they are to suffer from tinnitus at some stage in their lives. The hearing problem can be due to a defect in the outer or inner part of the ear, regardless of the reasoning of the hearing problem, tinnitus will occur in such individuals.

A brief history of tinnitus

Health concern related to tinnitus has spread over strata of general population. Ringing in the ears has been mentioned in texts from ancient histories. In 1931, Dr Thompson translated historical Babylonian medical texts; these texts were previously kept in the library of King Assurbanipal (668-626 BC) in

Nineveh (present day Iraq). These translations included 22 references to Tinnitus, described as whispering or ringing in the ears. Tinnitus studies have been the point of interest for more than five decades now and the research material related to tinnitus has been doubling every decade since 1950. A total of 67 papers were published before 1960 and 2 of these 67 were listed back in the 1880s (Hemming and Sexton). In the 1980s a total 109 papers were listed and 161 in 1990s. The count for the 1st decade of 21st century was 311 and 411 for 2010. Now more than 500 papers and scientific materials have been published each year. The number of basic research papers have now exceeded to more than 1000. Covering basic information, clinical statistics, management and critical research, all this research material has contributed a lot to build understanding and mechanism of the treatment for tinnitus.

Currently there is no pharmacological compound specifically authenticated for the medication of tinnitus; nonetheless, there are several products that are presently available for symptoms relief and minimize the indications that lead to severe forms of tinnitus and most of these drugs have been successfully tested in clinical trials. (One of these is 'Natural Quiet'.) Related disorders of tinnitus, like depression and anxiety, are pharmacologically treated in sufficient ratios with anti-depressants and other mood stimulants.

Definitions: Explanation of the various definitions of tinnitus in medical literature

Tinnitus is mostly defined as sensation of sound produced in the ears without any external source and stimulation. In another report from the Bioacoustics & Biomechanics (CHABA) committee on hearing proposed the definition of tinnitus as "a specific kind of noise that is generated and heard inside the human head". These two definitions are related to hearing hallucinations of schizophrenia. Schizophrenia is basically a neurotic disorder that is the difficulty of thought processing and deficit of typical emotional responses. Another definition of tinnitus says; "Tinnitus is an abnormal and unnatural type of sound that has no interaction to external source of stimulation".

All these definitions are based on several medical and historical evidences and the perception of tinnitus varies due to variable factors of external sounds. All patients of tinnitus perceive it as a sound entirely different from anything they have experienced from their external surroundings. A clinical study was conducted to demonstrate that the patients with tinnitus differentiate the ringing of tinnitus entirely different from other external sounds that they have experienced in the past.

Why there is no precise definition of tinnitus

A very common misconception related to Tinnitus is that most of the patients thought of it as a disease. However, tinnitus is a symptom and not a disease. Ringing ears are just like other common symptoms like fever, headache and pain. All diseases are primarily treated by lowering its symptoms, so the same method can be applied for managing tinnitus. Secondly, patients of tinnitus interpret their reasoning, their symptoms and environmental factors and ringing in the ears differently, that's why it has been difficult for clinicians to come up with a common definition of this illness. There are also several additional factors involved; the ringing in the ears can be the result of psychological issues as well as medical disorders such as chemical imbalance. Nonetheless, sometimes tinnitus can be the result of a side-effect of some medications under specific conditions. Tinnitus has been observed as a side effect in some psychiatric patients taking anti-depressants and mood stabilizers for their mental conditions.

Role of neurotransmitters in tinnitus

The chemical imbalance that we have previously talked about is due to neurotransmitters. These are the chemicals that are responsible for transmitting or forwarding information and instructions as signals. These signals are transmitted in the form of electrical pulses from a human's nervous system to the target cell, across a synapse. The release of neurotransmitters results in ease of intracellular and extracellular communications. There are several types of neurotransmitters that are classified on the basis of amino acids, monoamines and peptides. Nitric oxide, Somatostatin, Glutamate, Aspartate, GABA, Adrenaline, Acetyl choline and Serotonin are some major neurotransmitters in the human body.

The chemical disturbance or inadequate production of neurotransmitters can result in various psychotic disorders like stress, anxiety, mood variations, depression or even ringing in the ears. One particular neurotransmitter that has been associated with tinnitus is GABA (gamma amino butyric acid).

2 Understanding Tinnitus

Tinnitus is a very common term that seems to be innocuous but actually directs to a potentially disabling source that has harmed many but understood by few. Individuals often do not realise the severity of their adverse circumstance until they are so affected and come to a point where they can no longer help themselves. They are no longer in the shadow of peace and comfort and sometimes the reason can be very simple but beyond comprehension without external assistance. Tinnitus is a condition, a disorder, that needs to be understood and properly treated otherwise it will slip into a life gradually and will rob its meaning and source of satisfaction. This gradual loss is minor and imperceptible in the beginning, but eventually weighs so heavily that the sufferer's life becomes miserable.

Once the symptoms start to appear, then the course of tinnitus changes with the person and with the form of noises and ringing. It can last for days, weeks, months or years if left untreated. The risk of tinnitus is the same for males and females, adolescents, mid-lifers and old age persons. Nevertheless, the severity and ratio of prevalence alters in different age groups and working environments. If the reason of tinnitus is psychological, then females have more likely to get victimised than males and the same can be observed for old aged persons in comparison with youngsters and teenagers. This ratio has been reported in most of the countries regardless of working environment, exposure to loud noises, economic, racial or ethnic background.

Figure: 1 (Tinnitus Prevalence worldwide)

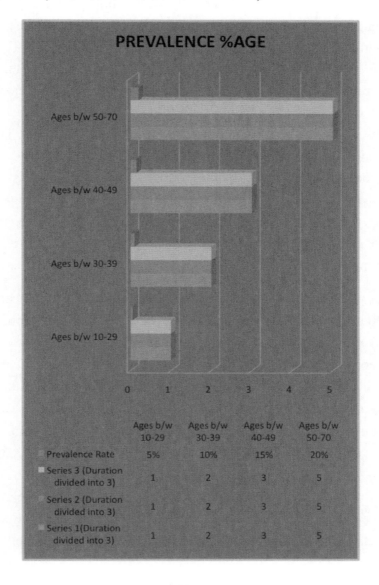

Cost of tinnitus

Some of the most creative, productive and influential individuals are included in the list of tinnitus sufferers. It is now understandable that the direct and indirect cost of this illness is getting higher and higher. A research study conducted by National Institute of Health of United States revealed that an estimated cost that the country is paying under victimisation of severe diseases like tinnitus, psychological and depressive disorders has increased to over 50 billion in a single year. These expenses include direct cost of treatment, reduced or lost productivity of tinnitus patients, absenteeism and disability payments. Although tinnitus does not always lead to such health hazards resulting in death, some individuals have been reported to attempt suicide under depression of their illness and hopelessness of their condition.

In America the prevalence rate is around 10% affecting nearly 30 million of the total population. These statistics are published by ATA (American Tinnitus Association).Thirteen million people have tinnitus without hearing loss and the highest prevalence ratio is present in ages of 65 to 84 years; Tinnitus patients reporting the impacts as 39% in hearing, 26% in concentration and 20% in sleep. Benefits of tinnitus treatment have been reported as; a) Hearing aids 34% and b) Music 30%. 40% of people reported that the experience of noises in the ears is >80% during a specific time of day or during each week. One very major issue observed that only a few patients felt relieved with their hearing aids and music therapies all of the time.

Noticeably, those patients who needed professional services for fitting their hearing aid using comprehensive fitting protocols benefited twice as much relief from their tinnitus. Whereas, those who didn't follow complete fitting protocols did not benefit as much.

Sergie Kochkin, Ph.D., from The Better Hearing Institute, Richard Tyler, Ph.D., from the University of Iowa, and Jennifer Born, American Tinnitus Association Director of Public Affairs and Tinnitus Today editor, collaborated to determine the prevalence of tinnitus in a nationally representative sample of more than 46,000 households - the largest survey of its kind.

Understanding the anatomy & physiology of the ear and the role of 'Stereocilia'

Anatomy of the Ear: *"The ear, or organ of hearing, is divisible into three parts: the external ear, the middle ear or tympanic cavity, and the internal ear or labyrinth.*

The external ear consists of the expanded portion named the auricula or pinna, and the external acoustic meatus. The former projects from the side of the head and serves to collect the vibrations of the air by which sound is produced; the latter leads inward from the bottom of the auricula and conducts the vibrations to the tympanic cavity.

The middle ear or tympanic cavity is an irregular, laterally compressed space within the temporal bone. It is filled with air, which is conveyed to it from the nasal part of the pharynx through the auditory tube. It contains a chain of movable bones, which connect its lateral to its medial wall, and serve to convey the vibrations communicated to the tympanic membrane across the cavity to the internal ear.

The internal ear is the essential part of the organ of hearing, receiving the ultimate distribution of the auditory nerve. It is called the labyrinth, from the complexity of its shape, and consists of two parts: the osseous labyrinth, a series of cavities within the petrous part of the temporal bone, and the membranous labyrinth, a series of communicating membranous sacs and ducts, contained within the body cavities.   (Gray's Anatomy, 20th Edition)

Constant exposure to loud noises, jet engine, rock concert, head or neck injuries, strong influencing earwax, ear infections and modifications can cause acute tinnitus. Accurate evaluation and the right treatment can result in resolution of tinnitus sounds. If the severity of tinnitus remains constant for more than 6 months then the situation is termed as 'Chronic Tinnitus'. Subjective tinnitus is commonly caused as a result of exposure to extreme noisy sounds like loud music, huge noises of heavy machinery and gunfire. Ringing noise is generated in the ears due to damage of Stereocilia within the cochlea.

Stereocilia

Clusters of hair-like addendums, which are called Stereocilia, reside in inner ear. When sound waves pass through the ears and hit their target hair cells, then these waves divert off the stereocilia, causing them to act in accordance to the power and tilt of the waves.

For example, a piano tune would create placid movement in the stereocilia, although heavy metal would induce hasty and sharper motion. This motion produces an electrochemical current that transmits a message from the sound waves with the help of auditory nerves to the brain.

Unusually, when we listen to loud noises, stereocilia become impaired. Then stereocilia gives false instructions to the auditory nerve cells. For instance, in rock concerts and fireworks' parades, it develops a resonant because the Stereocilia of inner ears have absolutely intermittent information and that's why we hear the wrong vibrations in the resonant of the head that we call Tinnitus.

Generally in its early stages, the impact of attack of noise-induced tinnitus is both alternative and sometimes even. Exposure to loud noises for a short period of time produces a mild form of tinnitus, but once the person affected is detached or driven away from the source of loud noises, then the effect of tinnitus reduces automatically. Thus, the sufferer can hear normally until exposed to the loud sound once again. This irregular pattern in tinnitus can be experienced periodically; usually it continues for months or even years with longer periods of ringing in the ear and eventually the noise in the ear becomes constant. Continuous exposure to loud noise can aggravate tinnitus and patients may perceive an increase in loudness and a change in pitch.

Loud noises can result in temporary hearing loss or generation of noises inside the head. The human nervous system receives sound waves through a process-vibration due to sound creating movement in hairs of each hair cell known as Stereocilia. Back and forth movement of hairs in stereocilia produces electrical impulses picked up by neurotransmitters that convey these signals to the brain as sound(s). These neurotransmitter molecules are triggered through basal end of hair cells that put in action the auditory neurons in CN VIII (8th cranial nerve). Extra hearing of sound (85 dB SPL or higher) results in Stereocilia bending more than normal and in this way sufferers perceive different kinds of ringing and noises in their heads or ears because loud noises instantly damage the hair cells that respond to high frequency sounds present in Stereocilia.

Recovery of Stereocilia damage depends upon its nature and frequency. If the damage is modest, then a person can get rid of ringing in the ears by recovering within hours up to a couple of days. Medical treatment and surgery of auditory system (stereocilia in the cochlea) can resolve the issue as well. If unfortunately, the exposure to loud noises is consistent and unavoidable and the damage can be severe and permanent, and tinnitus will become moderate to chronic. Exposures to something other than loud noises, like a disease or an accident, may cause damage to auditory nerve system and can also result in generation of tinnitus.

Understanding the different mechanisms of tinnitus

Clinicians and practitioners have proposed several mechanisms of tinnitus. At times debates about these mechanisms have turned into strenuous activity. Psychiatrists and medical experts have faced many challenges relating to their knowledge about tinnitus and its mechanisms. The most important factor of them all is to diagnose and monitor what is happening to the auditory system of the person suffering from tinnitus. Observations of tinnitus in both psychological and pathological ways are important. Just like related stress factor and neuroimaging function of the brain are supposed to be significant in determining the situation. There are two possible types of mechanisms 1) igniting or initiating point of tinnitus, 2) promoting or enhancing mechanisms. Such classification of mechanisms may not be conclusive but it will certainly help in the recognition and reorganising for diagnosis as well as treatments of tinnitus. Last but not least, understanding the human auditory system in detail, its complexity and its areas of possible disorders, can certainly improve the areas of methods of tinnitus surgeries, and the medications to prevent and treat tinnitus disorder.

Tinnitus and noise generation

The sound of tinnitus can be both real and imaginary. Noise generation and prevalence in childhood and adulthood is similar. By and large tinnitus is more prevalent in children who have hearing disorders and these disorders can either be sensor neural or conductive. The intensity of noise generation increases with increasing intensity of hearing impairments. Medically, tinnitus is a noise perception in one or both ears or in the head. These noises can be heard as ringing, whistling, roaring, hissing, clicking or chirping without any sound produced externally. The sound is completely subjective in tinnitus – a sound that can only be heard by the individual suffering with it.

Reference: Barbara Tabachnick Sanders,

ATA Director of Education Editor, Tinnitus Today

Theory 1 "Many clinicians have distinguished different forms of tinnitus on different basis. All of them have faced multiple challenges due to limited knowledge and understanding of tinnitus. One theory is that auditory mechanism should be examined to acknowledge what is happening in the auditory system of a human being with noises in the ear. Clinical trials and targeted studies of a tinnitus patient's hearing mechanism, should explain the specific way the auditory system of such patients actually works."

Theory 2 "One theory targets more specifically a certain part of auditory system that is called the Cochlea. It can also be described as a container of sensory cells of hearing. Cochlea damage can be a reason of tinnitus and hearing loss and in order to function properly cochlea needs proper blood supply.

Also, cochlea can result in consumption of high energy from blood supply to maintain perfect balance of its cochlea fluids. It is believed that hearing loss or noise generation in ears may depend on the vascular impairment location; cochlea sensory cells can be affected due to damage."

Many clinical studies have considered the relationship between tinnitus and other symptoms, like hearing difficulties or loss of hearing. Nonetheless, no clear evidence has been published to reveal the real cause of tinnitus. Some researchers have agreed that the initial cause of tinnitus can be hearing loss resulting from damage to the auditory nervous system. However, all patients of severe tinnitus are not victims of hearing loss, that's why it is unclear to indicate that tinnitus is directly linked to hearing loss.

3 Types of Tinnitus

Today, people all over the world are suffering from Tinnitus disorder. Everyone is looking for an answer to their illness. And, answers are always hidden in apparently insignificant knowledge of that particular disorder. Tinnitus is a phenomenon that is wrapped up in so many underlying complications and diseases. It is now mandatory to classify and gather as much information as possible on types of sounds and tinnitus. People with severe tinnitus may have difficulty in hearing, working, or even sleeping. Types of tinnitus are classed on different basis.

Breaking Tinnitus:

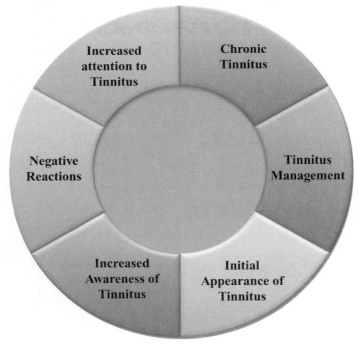

How many types of tinnitus?

According to the ability to be perceived by the external examiner, it can be distinguished as: Subjective Tinnitus, and Objective Tinnitus.

- In objective tinnitus, the sound is audible to the external examiner; it is also called 'pseudo-tinnitus'. It is caused by sound generated in the body that is then transmitted to the ears through conduction in body tissues. It is a rare type of tinnitus. Objective tinnitus can arise from muscle spasms that cause a click, or crackling sound around the middle ear. Pulsatile tinnitus could be objective in nature as it may result from increased blood turbulence, increased localised or generalised blood flow. But it could be the subjective phenomenon that results from altered awareness.

- In subjective tinnitus, only sufferers can hear the sound and it is most unusual. It is also called 'true tinnitus' or 'intrinsic tinnitus' and it is usually caused by an abnormal neural activity, and could be the side effect of certain medicines like NSAIDs and Antibiotics. It can also occur in result of benzodiazepine withdrawal. The causes of Subjective tinnitus include diseases like otology disorders that cause hearing loss. There are no subjective tests that can measure subjective tinnitus. Subjective tinnitus is not a disease, but a symptom that has a different underlying pathophysiology. It occurs with different severities and causes suffering that may affect social life to its worse. It consists of meaningless sounds that are not associated with any physical sound.

Classification based on the description of the patient includes:
- 'Tinnitus aurium' in which sound is in the ear,
- 'Tinnitus cerebri' in which sound is in the brain.

Description of the nature of tinnitus includes:
- low-pitched noise of sea
- high-pitched whistle
- roaring of machinery
- multiple sounds together resulting in complex sound

Classification according to associated phenomena includes:
- nature and type of hearing loss
- presence or absence of vestibular abnormalities
- the sounds generated in the inner ear

Classification according to the response treatment is also very important as Tinnitus is a symptom indicating an underlying disease so symptomatic treatment is the main kind that includes:
- response to masking
- response to medications
- treatment of underlying diseases and of psychological problems

Different types of Tinnitus can be differentiated according to life span that includes:
- acute tinnitus that lasts for less than 3 months

- sub-acute tinnitus that lasts between 4-6 months
- chronic tinnitus that lasts for more than 6 months

It could also be classified as Temporary tinnitus, and Permanent tinnitus. The main difference between them is the time scale within which they are experienced.

- Permanent tinnitus occurs frequently, and on a daily basis. There is no cure for permanent tinnitus, and patients try to habituate themselves to the sound or try some distraction therapy.

- Temporary tinnitus is usually the result of noise trauma and lasts between the time periods of a few hours to a few days. It is usually experienced when loud noise or music is heard in concerts or discos.

Tinnitus can also be classified according to the effects reported by the patients and this includes:
- 'Compensated Tinnitus'
- 'Decompensated Tinnitus'

In Compensated Tinnitus, the patient reports the sound that is bearable, and results in little or no psychological strain. The quality of life of the patient is not affected to a significant degree in this particular type. However in Decompensated Tinnitus, the sufferer hears sounds that are caused by the interference in the brain's hearing system. If emotions or stress exaggerates this interference then it will result in constant activation of the interference in sections of temporal lobe of the cortex. It is also called 'centralised tinnitus' and it works on the same principal as of 'phantom pain'. Tinnitus may occur to any possible severity ranging from acute to moderate to severe.

Tinnitus is also classified on the basis of Type of Sound as:
- Pulsatile Tinnitus
- Non-pulsatile Tinnitus

Pulsatile tinnitus

Pulsatile tinnitus is a rhythmic noise that has the same rate as the heart. It is checked by feeling the pulse and listening to the tinnitus at the same time. There are other types of tinnitus in which rhythm is present, but it is not synchronised with the pulse. It is the sound created by the ear canal, muscle movements near the ear or due to blood flow problems in face or neck vessels. It can be heard as sound of your pulse or contraction of the muscles. Another cause of pulsatile tinnitus is benign intracranial hypertension that is characterised by headaches and visual disturbance. During investigation of tinnitus patients, it is difficult to find any single reason as to the cause of tinnitus. Chances of finding a specific cause are greater with the Pulsatile Tinnitus than Non-pulsatile Tinnitus. It is investigated by stethoscope and ultrasound, CT, MRI, MRA, and CTA.

Other forms of Rhythmic tinnitus are rhythmic but not synchronised with the person's heartbeat. This type of tinnitus is due to the contraction of muscles in the middle ear. Malleus and stapes are the two small bones of the middle ear that are attached with two muscles named the tensor tympani and stapedius. Sometimes these muscles go into rhythmic contraction, a condition called Myoclonus. Rarely this rhythmic tinnitus can be caused by the contraction of a few muscles of the soft palate. Patulous Eustachian Tube Syndrome is another type of tinnitus. In this syndrome people experience the tinnitus that varies with their breathing. The Eustachian tube is the pressure balancing tube that runs from the back of the nose to inside the nose. It is normally shut, but if it becomes abnormally open then pressure changes due to breathing. The syndrome is due to excessive opening of this tube.

Non-pulsatile tinnitus

Non-Pulsatile Tinnitus is a continuous type of tinnitus. It is caused by a problem in the nerves that are required for the hearing process. The patients describe it as coming from inside the head and it is an auditory phantom phenomena resulting from auditory differentiation. Any lesion in the auditory track that results in altered functioning causes Non-pulsatile tinnitus.

Following are the causes of non-pulsatile tinnitus

Ménière's disease, Vestibular Schwannoma, micro-vascular compression, brain tumours etc.

Further classifications of Tinnitus are as follows:

Bruit: It is the term used when blood makes an unusual sound while flowing through an obstruction, i.e. turbulent flow. In bruit, patients complain of noise within the head that could be bubbling or pulsating. Bruit can be recorded by means of auscultation through microphone or the stethoscope as physically existing sound in the human skull and it is heard by the patients. Bruit can originate from the middle ear or the cause could be vascular in origin. Causes are middle ear inflammation, open Eustachian tube, arethroma, high blood pressure, scars or compressions.

Some crackling sounds are reported from arthritic, or mandibular joint disorders that are misinterpreted as tinnitus.

Endogenous tinnitus: Patients suffering with endogenous or maskable tinnitus, prefer covering it with external sounds. During the masking procedure, three types of zones are easily discriminated in the hearing field:
- Low-tone tinnitus (at and below 70Hz)
- Middle-frequency tinnitus (1 to 2kHz)
- High-frequency tinnitus (above 2kHz until 10kHz or even12kHz)

Low-tone tinnitus is commonly present with Ménière's disease. Middle-frequency tinnitus is frequently present in diseases such as otosclerosis. High-frequency tinnitus is related to stress, noise trauma, skull trauma, cardiovascular failure, neuromas, and with toxic events.

Exogenous tinnitus: In this, patients seek to avoid any outside noise. They report that the severity of tinnitus decreases as they go into the house or any other sound proof place. Patients suffering with Exogenous tinnitus cannot benefit from masking of the noises. Some physicians wrongly assume it as hyperacusis, but these patients don't hear well. Hearing aids are the first choice treatment for exogenous tinnitus as Hearing aids filter the incoming sound and clean sound signals so that they fit optimally into the existing hearing field of the individual. Some other methods are psychotherapy, pharmacotherapy, stress reduction and physiotherapy.

Relationship of tinnitus types and sound generating mechanisms

We have already discussed how different types of noises can be heard by a tinnitus patient. Now we need to understand a few other terminologies before we can understand the relationship between various types of tinnitus and their respective sound generating mechanisms.

Tinnitus masking

Tinnitus masking is the most common method in tinnitus therapy. Maskers generate signals that match with the tinnitus signals so they result in suppressing tinnitus sounds. The tinnitus masker substitutes the tinnitus sound with the less intrusive sound thus relieving the patient. Tinnitus masking leads to long-term changes in the brain; this process is called habituation. It reduces the tinnitus intensity and awareness of it and that comes under Tinnitus Retaining Therapy.

Dr Jack Vernon is one of the founders of the American Tinnitus Association. As a tinnitus patient too he observed and synthesised the sound of falling water, which is an effective masker of tinnitus. Today tinnitus maskers range from CD, MP3, noise generators, wearable devices and hearing aids.

Wearable maskers: The first sound generator was added to a hearing aid to mask tinnitus and for external sound amplification in 1974. They are known as combination devices or wearable sound generators (WSG). They are used by the patients who need masking around the clock. WSGs cannot reproduce high frequency sound that is required by the Tinnitus patient so they are not very effective. So here there is a need to improve wearable hearing aid devices. Other wearable maskers include Neuromonics, Tinnitus Phase-Out and TRT.

Neuromonics: This is a six-month long therapy that results in reduced tinnitus awareness and minimises the impact of tinnitus on patient's life. The process uses sound generating devices that deliver neutral sounds that are designed to match the tinnitus profile of patients.

Tinnitus phase-out: It works on the principle that every sound has an opposing sound which completely neutralises each other's effect. In this system, sound pattern is matched with the specific pitch of the patient and volume levels. Tinnitus Phase-Out™ system is simple, easy to use, and requires no wearable devices.

Tinnitus retaining therapy (TRT): Is a form of habituation therapy that uses counselling to explain to the patients that tinnitus retaining and sound enrichment can minimize the impact of Tinnitus. It uses sound generators frequently to provide the background noise level.

Masking CDs and sound generators: These are the most effective ways to mask tinnitus without the WSG fitting, using the following types of noise:

- **White noise** is the most common noise used to mask tinnitus for example ringing sound. It is analogous to white light and is a great masker as it contains all frequencies of sound in equal proportions, so patients find it a relaxing sound. It blocks the distracting sounds and helps in improving concentration.

Highest frequencies could be harsh to the ears so other shades of noise are also used as they are not harsh e.g. pink and brown noise.

- **Pink noise** is a more natural sound for masking as highest frequencies have been filtered out, so it is more comfortable to the ears.

- **Brown noise** is the sound with lower frequency than white and pink noise so it is most effective for masking low frequency tinnitus sounds such as rumbles or roars. It is not suitable for ringing tinnitus. Brown noise is similar to the distant sound of the sea.

There are many **sound generators** that have range of noise and natural sound. The speakers cannot reproduce highest frequencies so they cannot mask high pitched tinnitus tones. So

Tinnitus Masking CDs are more effective. Masking tapes are uncommon today because of high frequency output, CDs have sampling rates 44.1 kHz can reach 20 kHz.

Nature sounds are more relaxing and enjoyable among people; white, pink and brown noises are the simple synthetic versions of water as they have similar frequencies. The sound is identical to the noise of waves of the sea. Some nature sounds are distracting such as bird calls.

Explanation of different types of sounds of tinnitus

They could be of different types, but it will fall usually within categories of ringing, buzzing, hissing, whooshing, screeching, whistling and static, cricket, ocean waves, clicking, music or even a pulsing beat. The volume of the tinnitus sound varies from very soft to extremely loud. Buzzing and ringing are reported often by the tinnitus sufferers as 'come and go'. **Buzzing** is really annoying and sometimes disturbs the concentration of the sufferer at work or even at sleep time and it is the second common type of tinnitus sound. Tinnitus **ringing** sound just resembles the bell ringing in church. It could be the 'come and go' type, or sometimes it is permanent. This can affect one ear or both depending upon the severity of the tinnitus. The severity of tinnitus will depend on the cause of your tinnitus. The **hissing** type of tinnitus sound is treatable; it resembles the sound produced during making tea. Any type of tinnitus sound can be treated if we know the cause behind it and if the cause is treatable then tinnitus sound can be treated as well. Otherwise if there is more than one complication behind the tinnitus, the cure will be difficult or impossible. **Whistling or roaring** type tinnitus sound is the worst type as it destroys your social life. It basically sounds like a roar that is associated with bad blood flow. This sound has many different causes and it is the rarer type of tinnitus sounds. It is not treatable as it has so many causes that may complex the situation. **Pulsatile (pulsing beat)** sound is synchronised with person's heart beat and it is rhythmic to the pulse. However some people hear their tinnitus as music or songs; these are called 'musical-hallucination' or 'auditory imagery'. They are less common than usual tinnitus sounds and may range from simple tones to songs.

4 Causes of Tinnitus

There are several causes to this disorder. One of the most common causes of tinnitus is the disturbance of signals to the auditory system. This incident may occur due to three reasons; cochlear malfunction, conductive hearing loss or abnormality of the auditory nerve. The most common triggers of the tinnitus include; exposure of ears to loud sounds, intake and usage of various drugs, feeling emotional, work stress, head injury and various kinds of ear conditions including infections and diseases. These triggers are explained in detail in the following paragraphs.

Exposure to loud noises

The most frequent cause of tinnitus is exposure to loud noises. An explanation for this is that excessive noise exposure is known to be one of the major factors that affect the auditory system at various levels causing hearing loss and tinnitus. When a person is near to loud noises for a long period of time then he is likely to develop tinnitus.

In our everyday life, people are facing greater threats due to increasing level of noise pollution in our environment and surroundings. Various noises like traffic and recreational noises make it even worse for the patients of tinnitus. Leisure activities may also be an additional trigger to tinnitus. This includes anything from the extensive use of MP3 players and iPods to high intensity musical instruments. In up to 90% of people, noise-induced hearing loss is the main cause of tinnitus. Some people whose jobs are around loud music have a greater risk of getting tinnitus, for example rock musicians, pilots, street-repair workers, carpenters, and landscapers. A single exposure to such a sudden, intensely loud noise can also cause tinnitus. Consequences of noise exposure occur both gradually or unexpectedly.

Loud noise effects on the cochlea

The cochlea is a spiral-shaped organ in the inner ear, so the noise causes a permanent loss of the sound-sensitive cells of the cochlea. People want to listen to loud music, but they don't realise that continued exposure to loud noises may result in the loss of their hearing ability. Such an effect can also put individuals in a position where there are maximum chances of worsening of the tinnitus.

Loud noise affects in a manner that it creates impact on the inner ear of the cochlea. Noise levels louder than normal levels can damage parts of our inner ears called hair cells. Inside the cochlea these hair cells are present. Hair cells work as the sentinel of our hearing; when sound waves strike these hair cells, they convert them into electrical currents then the auditory nerves carry them to the brain. There is no other striking medium inside the inner ear to which sound waves hit.

Side effect of medication

The second most common cause of tinnitus is from the intake of various forms of prescribed and self-medicated drugs. Currently, hundreds of these types of drugs are in common use. Medications that can increase intensity of tinnitus include antibiotics, anaesthetics (painkillers, analgesics, sedatives), diuretics, anti-anxiety and anti-depression drugs, anti-malarial medications, anti-cancer drugs and blood pressure controlling medications.

Many drugs may cause and increase the incidence of tinnitus and depending on the dose of these drugs it could be temporary or permanent. Higher doses of these medications result in severe forms of tinnitus. The side effects caused by medication may vary from person to person.

Antibiotics are those drugs prescribed by the physicians specifically to increase the ability of the humans' immune system that fight against bacterial infections. Fighting a wide range of bacteria, a broad spectrum of antibiotics is now available. Unfortunately, the regular antibiotics that are most commonly used today are known to be affective against only a particular symptom. Some types of antibiotics destroy bacteria while other types become a barrier in their reproduction cycle and stop reproducing. Antibiotics are not effective for viral infections. Various antibiotics are considered to be responsible for the production of tinnitus in affected people, such as erythromycin, kanamycin, neomycin, gentamicin, streptomycin, deoxycyclinex, chloramphenicol, vancomycin and polymyxin B. Some medications/drugs can trigger tinnitus by direct toxicity to the ear. This direct toxicity is called ototoxicity. Gentamicin is an antibiotic that belongs to a class of drugs called aminoglycosides. Aminoglycosides can cause tinnitus by direct toxicity. So, this class of antibiotics is prominent for its ototoxicity. However, many medications cause tinnitus through adverse side effects in which the production mechanism of tinnitus is not known.

Anti-cancer drugs: Anti-cancer drugs whose side effects can stimulate tinnitus include Bleomycin, Cisplatinum, Carboplatinum, Methotrexate, Nitrogen mustard and Vinblastin.

Anti-malarial medications: Chloroquine and Hydroxychloroquine drugs can cause tinnitus.

Diuretics: Acetazolamide, Bumetanide, Clorothalidone, Ethacrynic acid, Hydrochlorthiazide, Methylchlorthizide.

Anaesthetics: Anaesthetics consist of painkillers, analgesics and sedatives. These anaesthetics include Bupivacain, Lidocaine and tetracain which may trigger tinnitus.

Non-steroidal anti-inflammatory drugs (NSAIDS): Non-Steroidal anti-inflammatory drugs can increase the chances of tinnitus. In this class, aspirin is the main drug which can cause severe tinnitus.

Aspirin: Aspirin is also called acetylsalicylic acid. Aspirin is an over-the-counter medication that can be found combined with many prescriptions. Excessive use of aspirin is a common cause of tinnitus and stopping its use will make it go away. Other drugs having the potential of causing tinnitus include Acematacine, Diclofenac, Diflunisal, Fenoprofen, Ibuprofen, Indomethacin, Methyl salicylates, Naproxen, D-Penicilliami and Phenylbutazone.

Anti-depressants: Anti-depressant drugs may worsen tinnitus. Zoloft and celexa are two main anti-depressants that can cause tinnitus.

Zoloft: Zoloft is also called sertraline. This prescribed medicine belongs to a class of antidepressants known as selective serotonin reuptake inhibitors (SSRI). Approximately 1% to 10% of patients using sertraline have experienced tinnitus of varying severities.

Celexa: Celexa is also called citalopram. This prescribed medicine also belongs to a class of antidepressants known as selective serotonin reuptake inhibitors (SSRI). Tinnitus occurs as an adverse effect once Celexa is discontinued.

Ear or head injury

Our auditory system is a complicated network and highly sensitive to disturbance. If an injury takes place, hair cells of the cochlea can be permanently destroyed which results in the suppression of sound.

Ear or head injury is often associated with a severe kind of tinnitus. Tinnitus is a common problem associated with both severe head injury to mild head injury. An attack of tinnitus is more severe if a person has pre-existing hearing loss. Head traumas cause tinnitus by discharging excessive fluid in the middle and inner ear. Head trauma causes bleeding on the external part of the brain and brain stem. In turn, this bleeding triggers to destroy the cochlea which is the inner ear. The cochlea is a sensitive part that consists of membranes and sacs filled with different fluids. If these sacs rupture due to an injury, fluid leaks and this can cause hearing loss and tinnitus. When the inner ear is injured, it may deliver wrong messages to the brain and we know these false connections are amplified in the brain, resulting in the worsening of tinnitus sounds.

Diseases of the ear

Outer ear disorders: Ear wax, ear drum affected by hairs and pierced ears can stimulate the loss of hearing and cause tinnitus.

Middle ear disorders: Fluid accumulation, otosclerosis, tumours, negative pressure from Eustachian tube, eustachian tube blockage due to allergies or viruses and foreign objects in the ear can also cause tinnitus.

Inner ear disorders: Hearing loss due to loud noise exposure, ageing and Ménière's disease are often associated with tinnitus.

Hearing loss and related tinnitus often occurs due to the dysfunction of the organs of the vestibular system. Some vestibular disorders related with tinnitus involve Ménière's disease. It is an inner ear disorder that can cause hearing loss, tinnitus and a feeling of pressure deep inside the ear. This syndrome appears to be the result of the abnormal amount or composition of fluid in the inner ear.

Ear infections

Hearing in humans is highly sensitive to infection. Certain ear infections can also cause tinnitus. For example, many people along with children suffer from tinnitus due to middle ear infections (otitis media) or sinus infections. Middle ear problems are most commonly related to infections. Commonly, once the infection clears up the tinnitus will reduce and gradually diminishes. Other diseases of the ear that can cause tinnitus involve the accumulation of calcium on small bones of the middle ear. This condition is called otosclerosis and is induced by certain types of viral infections. Occurrence of tinnitus increases due to otosclerosis.

Ear wax blockage: When there is a temporary conductive hearing loss due to ear infection or due to blockage of the ear with wax it may cause tinnitus. The ear canal is typically considered part of the outer ear. Hair and ear wax is produced in the outer section of the ear canal. It protects the ear from dirt, dust and bacteria, so it helps to prevents infection. Wax is an important and natural secretion found in the ear. It protects the ear against dust, dirt and bacteria, and it helps to prevent infection. Wax, or cerumen as it is also known, is composed of epithelium (skin cells), dust and oily secretions from the sebaceous and ceruminous glands in the ear canal. These secretions lubricate the ear canal and prevent it from becoming too dry. The composition of wax varies from person to person depending on their eating habits, their ages and environmental factors also play a vital role.

When water enters the ear due to any reason this may cause expansion of wax in the ear giving a perception of 'blockage' in the ear. This condition increases the rate of developing tinnitus.

Effect of different types of stress on tinnitus

Stress is a natural response to outside stimulus and its consequences are both positive and negative. Stress has been strongly linked to the development of temporary and permanent tinnitus. Many stress factors such as job stress, economic hurdles, mental pressure during preparation of exams and many more countless reasons can be potential sources. Also, these can contribute toward worsening tinnitus as when our body is under stress, many changes can take place in our body. For example, physical, chemical and hormonal changes can occur and disturb our mechanical balance. Such an imbalance can lead to many complications like blood vessels constriction and reduced circulations, increased heart rate and breathing rate and increased blood pressure. Stress always attacks us at our weakest point, whether mental or physical and prolonged exposure to stress may create many problems.

Stress is a significant factor in inducing tinnitus. Tension or stress stimulates the fight or flight systems of our body which produces a great deal of pressure on blood flow, nerves and body heat. This induced pressure and stress then reaches at their target point that is the inner ear. Here this pressure damages the cochlea which results in loss of hearing and tinnitus. Mostly, this type of tinnitus is temporary. Uncontrolled stress, tension and anxiety often make tinnitus worse and vice versa.

Emotional stress

Emotional stress includes depression, anxiety, sadness and grief which can contribute to gradual tinnitus build-up. Depressed people are affected with tinnitus more easily as compared to those who are not depressed. When emotional stress is constant and prolonged, such as anxiety and depression, it can provoke tinnitus. Continued exposure to stress will make the tinnitus noises much louder than they would be in a relaxed form. The hypothalamus and other parts of the brain like pituitary fossa, brain stem and the ventricular systems take part in promoting tinnitus. The hypothalamus and the structures in the brain that are under its control are important for producing vital chemicals. These chemicals are essential for our body to work normally. Prolonged exposure to stress, sudden shock, anxiety and grief have a great influence on hypothalamus. Then, the hypothalamus does not work properly and in return those essential chemicals are not produced by the hypothalamus - this may be a leading cause of tinnitus.

Job stress

Job stress is a seriously harmful and inevitable physical and emotional response that occurs when the requirements of the job do not match the capabilities, resources, or needs of the worker. Sometimes an individual finds it very difficult to perform at a certain level due to inability and inconsistency. All such situations can lead an individual to the point of desperation.

Many practitioners believe that certain types and amounts of stress are handy for us to perform efficiently. Sometimes pressure can make us realise the importance of the task and that can bring out our hidden abilities to our knowledge. Nonetheless, too much stress or being under stress for too long is not good with regard to physical and mental health and to some extent can also create additional disadvantages. Some people are very good at handling domestic and professional pressure and such individuals known to handle stress are found to have a low percentage of getting tinnitus. In comparison, those persons who do not know how to handle their circumstances and perform accordingly under stress, have a higher probability of getting tinnitus. Job stress can lead to poor health and even mental disabilities. Mental and physical issues may include, low self-esteem, hopelessness, helplessness, isolation, inability to perform high energy tasks, physical imbalance and tinnitus.

Job stress appears in various forms and affects our mind and body in different ways. Some professionals have a stressful nature which can contribute to tinnitus causation. Existing tinnitus increases in its intensiveness, and slows down coping systems in individuals of this category. It is possible when the autonomic nervous system is affected because of this.

Major stress comes from having too much work, not enough work or doing the type of work in which we are not interested. Miscommunications and misunderstandings among bosses and co-workers can also provoke job stress. We can get more stressed if we have too much work to do and giving more time to our professional duties can disturb domestic lifestyle. Additional adjustments to perform new tasks can also lead to a stressful condition and may also cause tinnitus.

Other possible causes

There are other possible conditions that can trigger tinnitus. Such as allergies, attack of sinus infection or cold, Lyme disease, fibromyalgia, diabetes, hormonal changes, deficiency of cerebrospinal fluid, vitamin depletion and intake of specific kind of foods. These specific kinds of foods includes grain-based spirits and red wine and can cause or increase tinnitus. In some people excessive amounts of alcohol or caffeine intake and smoking cigarettes can aggravate tinnitus.

5 Living with Tinnitus

Tinnitus is a medical anomaly in which the affected person hears different types of high as well as low pitched sounds. These sounds do not occur from outside of the body but the patient often feels that they originate from an outside source. Whilst the person may not have any hearing problems and he or she may seem perfectly normal and healthy, this condition can affect their daily life and hamper their ability to perform normally in society.

The word **tinnitus** has a Latin origin and its meaning is **ringing**. The word ringing is associated with the condition in which bell rings are usually heard in the ear. Tinnitus can occur because of many reasons:

- wax build up
- nasal allergies
- ear infections
- heavy medication
- stress
- foreign objects entering the ear
- disseminated sclerosis
- remaining in silence or in a loud noise area for a long time

One or both ears can be affected by tinnitus. The sounds that can be experienced may include high pitched shriek sounds, electric buzzes, humming, tings, whining and many other such noises/sounds. Tinnitus is described as worse at night because the external sounds commonly heard during the day help in masking the tinnitus sounds but at night it's different story.

This condition affects about one in six people as found in the scientific surveys. Most people aren't bothered if the sounds only last for about five minutes. It is more common for people above 50 years of age - surprisingly females are more affected than males and approximately half of the tinnitus sufferers experience it in one ear. People who face this phenomenon have anxiety attacks, get angry at minor problems and feel upset about their condition.

In order for this class of people to lead a prosperous and contented life they have to adjust with the problem. The first step would be to accept and move on - this is the foremost step and start of a new life. Secondly, the focus should be anger and anxiety management; anger eats you away like rust and it keeps you in a deep void making you virtually a silly burden on the society. Try to make people comfortable around you by not letting them know about your condition. This will help others get a good image of you and make you bolder and more confident in your daily routine.

One thing a sufferer needs to understand is that any medical condition whether cancer, tuberculosis or malaria needs time and effort to heal, and the same for tinnitus. It will take time to cure or manage the condition and this effort will make the person strong and wilful to fight off this disability for the better of all.

Common symptoms

Tinnitus can have several implications for the individual; it can be mere nuisance or it can cause major suffering and problems like insomnia, anxiety or panic attacks, depression and different types of phobias. Tinnitus may present itself as a group of ghostly sensations. These sensations are not disorders but symptoms of different kinds of anomalies that include the changes in neuroplasticity. Now we will discuss these symptoms in detail.

Sleeping problems (insomnia)

Scientific research shows that people who have tinnitus disorder are found to have problems during sleep like irregular leg movements and sleep apnoea. Sleep apnoea denotes to a condition in which instances of low breathing and sometimes pauses in breathing also occur. The pause can last from few seconds (mainly up to 10 seconds) to several minutes. These episodes can severely disrupt normal healthy sleep with the person becoming an insomniac at a later stage. Sleep is a major disorder in a tinnitus patient and over 70% people suffer from insomnia due to it. Sleep problems are not restricted to adults as reports indicate that more than 80% of children have complained of disturbed sleep due to tinnitus. However it is not conclusive that all suffers of tinnitus have sleep problems.

Although a lot of research into tinnitus leads to insomnia as a major symptom, a thorough analysis of this factor is yet to be done, to frame it more appropriately in the field of medicine.

Clinical reports suggest that sleepless nights are not directly linked with tinnitus but correspond to usual awakenings. The main cause of insomnia among tinnitus patients is the anxiety associated with tinnitus rather than with tinnitus itself.

In spite of the importance of sleep disorder in this condition, it has been ruled out as a direct cause, rather it is an interlinked phenomena proved by research.

Problem in concentration

Concentration is a big issue for a tinnitus sufferer. Lack of concentration is often a great despair. A patient usually has problems in concentrating on academic studies, calculations and cognitive processing. Two aspects of should be considered in a tinnitus patient are:
  • material of a person's thought
  • the ability to concentrate on things

The material aspect denotes a person's unique personality. This will affect the behaviour that a person carrying the tinnitus disorder will exhibit in society. Some people will be calm, some depressed and anxious and others can even have neutral thoughts. Studies have shown that thought processes have shown agony, despair, hopelessness, loss of belief and seem to incline more towards silence and wanting peace. All these factors directly or indirectly affect a person's cognitive process whilst disrupting concentration like a normal individual.

The second aspect is the ability to concentrate on things of importance like family, work and friends - these have been partially or permanently paralysed due to tinnitus. People who complain about their disability have reported to be more preoccupied in thinking about tinnitus and are more unproductive in mental skills.

Depression

Depression and tinnitus go together head-to-head. People who are severely affected by tinnitus often complain of depression and anxiety. Depression is related to subjective tinnitus and is likely to increase other problems like sleepless nights, loss of hunger, feeling of depravity and lack of social interaction. Tinnitus acts as an impetus which promotes psychiatric disorders in individuals as being opposed to a principle agent.

Major depressive disorder or (MDD) is also linked with tinnitus but some studies have shown that half of the depression patients had MDD prior to tinnitus development.

Studies also suggest that some patients who are suffering from tinnitus or depression are likely to have the other respective disorder as well and vice versa if they are not treated in time.

Tinnitus and relationships

Limited studies have been carried out on the impact of tinnitus on relationships. There is a possibility that family relations are affected by a person's condition. Spouse and children are equally affected and are subjected to different behavioural attitudes by a tinnitus sufferer. The kind of response can vary from person to person, for instance, if a spouse provides love and attention to the patient he/she may unintentionally be amplifying the patient's condition, whereas the spouse who ignores the aggressive behaviour may reduce the overall severity of the condition whilst improving his/her functionality. Tinnitus patients express their distress via various absurd behaviours. This also affects the children's psychological health and they are unable to communicate effectively with both parents. Sometimes children are a big moral support in helping a parent to cope with the problem as they become a reason and a motivation to live happily.

Tinnitus can also become a source of disrupted marriages and dysfunctional family structure. It is seen that the tinnitus affected patients get a better recovery rate if they are cared for within the family and by friends.

Work related issues

An individual's ability to work or carry out tasks easily is badly disrupted after having any type of disability. This is true for tinnitus patients; they are severely affected by this problem. Studies suggest that about 40 % of people having this disability, face difficulty in keeping up with their work commitments. A person may or may not inform his/her employer about their specific condition and keep it to themselves for several reasons and they fear that the person on the other end will not understand the problem, or the fear of losing the job or the fear of being a laughing stock among colleagues.

Modern telecommunication jobs particularly those involving

extensive use of headphones are directly associated with tinnitus and other hearing disorders. Workers in a call centre have an increased risk of getting tinnitus (30-40%).

Very few research literatures explain the obstruction that is caused by tinnitus on the ability of people to work, for instance, jobs that require precision hearing ability, like playing a musical instrument or singing. People will sometimes conceal the facts about their condition and keep performing their daily life tasks without anyone even knowing it. Jobs that require less concentration can be easily carried out by such individuals. Tinnitus-affected people can live normally by adopting coping strategies and addressing their fellow workers about their problem to lessen the impact they might have by not telling at all.

Environmental factors

Tinnitus can also be caused by environmental factors:

- Loud noises like music and heavy machinery sounds - a person having preliminary stage tinnitus can be affected by such exposure. People who work at factories or who play loud music may develop hearing loss symptoms. This hearing loss can equate to a gradual shift to tinnitus.

- A change in air pressure can also cause tinnitus; this is associated with barometric (air) pressure change. Travelling in an aeroplane or visiting a high mountainous area indicate an air pressure change and a person might experience clogged ears or ringing bells in one or both ears.

- Weather can also have an impact on tinnitus; wet weather accommodates moisture build up in the ear canal that when frozen by cold weather, is sure to promote bacterial activity. This can be prevented by covering the ears or using ear plugs.

- Ear wax can also cause trouble in some instances. Wax build up in the ear canal can cause agonizing discomfort to the individual and electrical buzzing like sound. Regular cleaning of ears performed by a professional is helpful in overcoming tinnitus.

Tinnitus counselling

Tinnitus is a condition believed by many to be incurable; there is nothing that can be done about. But this is not entirely true as the effect of tinnitus on a person can be lessened by proper management and medical, nutritional and psychological therapies like counselling.

Counselling is recommended for people who are diagnosed with tinnitus. People who face a mild form of tinnitus just need reassurance and some education to overcome their problem. Consultation from a professional audiologist is beneficial in this regard. People who are severely affected by tinnitus may need extra sessions with an audiologist. Several types of counselling available for a tinnitus patient:

Lay counselling

Lay counselling involves not a professional counsellor but a person who has some experience dealing with tinnitus. It may help many people who are nervous about going to a professional and open up to them. Lay counselling may include members of some NGO who run a self-help group. Lay counselling can be carried out face-to-face or through other mediums such as telephone, internet, video conferencing.

Private counselling

Private counselling involves a person who works independently or practices counselling in any medical or psychological organization. Such counsellors may or may not have professional training but they must be recognized by concerned authorities. It is not necessary for a private counsellor to be a tinnitus expert, but it can help to reduce the effect of tinnitus by easing the other complications that cause tinnitus like stress, anxiety, fear etc. Private counselling can be free or may be charged depending on the organization.

Group counselling

Group counselling includes more than one person suffering from tinnitus. Group counselling requires many sessions and it may involve one or more therapists.

A group session of people having tinnitus is thought to be more effective as it means that they can freely discuss their issues with other members and help themselves and others at the same time. These sessions help the participants deal and manage with their conditions more easily.

Medical counselling

Medical counselling is termed as professional help. An ENT (Ear Nose Throat) specialist will deliver the counselling to a tinnitus patient in his/her clinic. This sort of counselling includes other professionals in a session such as an audiologist. The success rate is quite high in medical counselling; patients are taught how to overcome their everyday obstacles through training psychotherapy.

Taking responsibility / lifestyle modification

Tinnitus used to be a non-curable condition as only management and lifestyle modification measures were considered helpful for the patient in the long run. The main aim of modification was to adjust the affected person with the everyday tasks without getting irritated with the condition.

An efficacious management plan can still be formulated to help the tinnitus patient after the availability of newer effective treatments; the plan can include the following:

- a clear and detailed analysis of the patients' health and psychosocial profile

- sessions of interviews between patient and clinical expert to understand the condition better

- a substantial amount of time spent with the patient (several hours at a time) for a better understanding include family members, parents, spouses and friends during the treatment process

After these conditions are met, the severity of tinnitus is a very important aspect that needs to be determined. Before the suggestions of lifestyle modification are proposed, a simple questionnaire consisting of three core information blocks, i.e. hearing, health and history, has to be completed by each patient to identify the severity of the tinnitus.

After the completion of the above steps, the clinical expert will spend some more time with the patient. This session will serve several important goals.

- an interview is important in a sense that the patient opens up to the physician one-on-one or in a group and it helps both of them to get together and feel comfortable with each other

- the session will help the patient to explain the questionnaire responses and gives the opportunity to the physician to ask additional questions of importance

- if family members, relatives and friends are joining the session, they can give important input on the patients' history of the disease, lifestyle and social activities

- discussion on specific problem areas with the patient

- suggestions on tinnitus combating strategies, protocols

and apparatus

- selective tinnitus treatments and management procedures for specific tinnitus condition are beneficial

Recommendation on lifestyle changes

With the review of patients' clinical history, lifestyle and work environment, the physician can now give recommendations to the patient on how to manage their lifestyle with tinnitus.

Changing patients' perceptions and expectations

Before a conventional physician starts the treatment of the patient, he/she is informed in writing that they cannot cure tinnitus. The aim of the therapy is to minimize and alleviate the agony a person faces during his/her daily life engagements. However it is important that the patient is given hope and not simply demoralized from the start. It is seen in cases that several patients having acute tinnitus have recovered by management strategies. It has been recorded in some observations that the patients who try to suppress their tinnitus are more severely affected by its ill effects. People are seen praying that their tinnitus might go away or seen running away from it. Unfortunately, they are the worst affected by it. Life for them is a daily struggle and nothing seems to be going their way. Such people are often deeply sunk into depression, anxiety and severe tinnitus. People who have some control over their thoughts can have better coping ability.

Improved sleep patterns

People who experience insomnia or lack of sleep often complain more about severe tinnitus than the patients who take proper and longer sleep. Improved sleep practice can minimize the intensity of tinnitus greatly. Some common remedies are:

- pleasant sounds introduced into the patient's bedroom. For this purpose sound generators are available that are often embedded with mattresses pillows; these sound generators play soothing sounds like the ocean waves and dripping raindrops

- medications should be improvised to help patient sleep better

- sleeping pills should be strictly used on prescription by the concerned doctor; it is not necessary to take the pills at every sleep

- patients should look forward to activities that can alleviate stress and relax the body

- special recommendations should be followed provided by the national sleep foundation

- if the condition of sleeplessness continues the patient should contact specialized sleeping disorder treatment facilities for comprehensive treatment

Some patients complain that even after getting enough sleep they still feel like they have been awake all night and tired. It is recommended by clinical experts that a thorough physical examination should be given by the physician including thyroid function, blood tests and haemoglobin concentration test.

Reduced anxiety

The severity of tinnitus is correlated to the level of anxiety that a patient faces. Like other psychological problems anxiety is also related to depression, lagging in communication, employment and social problems. Patients who exhibit continued anxiety symptoms are recommended to visit a psychiatrist and get evaluated. It is preferred that they visit the one who specializes in anxiety and stress related management. Patients may also benefit from registered therapeutic experts and counsellors who can guide them on soul and mind relaxation and stress relieve therapies. Some steps to reduce anxiety are:

- anxiety can be reduced by improvising some distraction mechanism which can help the patient to get his/her mind of the things of worry, for example exercising, yoga or talking to someone on the phone, indulging in a hobby

- reducing your anxiety by patting your pet or taking a warm bath and relaxing afterwards is a good choice

- people having anxiety attacks are recommended to visit a registered therapist and take professional help for learning anxiety reduction techniques

- drink lots of fluids, mostly water and go for morning

walks; there is no medicinal cure to relieve anxiety, it is only through anxiety management strategies that one can feel at ease

What you eat matters

There is a famous saying 'You are what you eat'. It is totally true because the health of a person entirely depends on their dietary intake. Studies suggest that by reducing the intake of coffee there was no significant relief in tinnitus, however there was less than 10 % people who faced severe tinnitus after taking caffeinated edibles. So statistically speaking a tinnitus patient can keep on taking their favourite caffeinated beverage and chocolates. Some patients report that they feel loudness of their tinnitus when they consume products containing lactose, sucrose and sodium. In light of this, the therapists ask the patients to give up these products on experimental temporary basis to decide whether they cause the problem or if it is all in the mind.

Supplements

Supplements are used by people to enhance their overall physical and mental potential. However, until very recently there were no specific dietary supplements that could help reduce tinnitus severity. Patients are now advised to take one or two multi-vitamin capsules/tablets every day after breakfast, i.e. 'Natural Quiet'. This might not help to lessen the tinnitus severity but it can improve the overall health of a patient and help to maintain the general health of the auditory system. The right combination of vitamins and herbs can produce miraculous results in tinnitus patients. People who are healthy can think better and can have greater control over their condition. A greater approach and positive thinking can help to reduce the severity of tinnitus and in time can eliminate all the symptoms.

Alcohol and narcotics

If alcohol and narcotics are used in small quantities it doesn't seem to affect tinnitus sufferers. Studies suggest that a drink or a smoke once in a while helps the patient to relax and does not affect tinnitus. A person overdoses on alcohol and narcotics will feel heavy headed and complain of increased tinnitus severity; this can be therefore eliminated by low to moderate usage. Using drugs of any sort to alleviate pain and used as a sleep aider, is not recommended because it can disturb the metabolism causing tinnitus and discomfort to the patient.

Exercise

Patients often avoid rigorous physical activities such as exercise; they complain that exercise increases their tinnitus. This type of tinnitus is temporary and associated with exertion that increases the blood flow in the arteries. The benefits of exercise outweigh the more temporary tinnitus, so it is recommended that patients should exercise regularly for health benefits such as better cardiovascular health, better physical health, increased sleep and stress reduction.

Self-modification

Patients describe that when they are busy at work or any other activity they are less bothered by tinnitus, even if they don't have a job. More people should indulge in activities and hobbies to take their mind off thinking about tinnitus. The activities such as an employment can help create self-responsibility in the person and hobbies can take their mind off dull lifestyles and turn things around him/her vibrant.

Cultivation of relationships

Personal relationships are severely affected by any mental or physical disorder. The same is for tinnitus; a tinnitus patient suffers heavily due to his/her condition. A person may avoid socialization because of noisy environments. Tinnitus therapists can encourage the affected people to make more social relations and cultivate friendships. The tinnitus patients who have supportive social structure i.e. family, friends and colleagues have better chances of successful treatment and management of their condition. It is also important for a person's spouse since he/she is the closest to help and support the patient at times of a tinnitus attack.

6 Importance of Accurate Diagnosis of Tinnitus

The importance of an accurate diagnosis is sometimes very difficult to understand. Both patients and medical professionals frequently fail to understand the exact severity of the tinnitus due to this misunderstanding. Although the lack of understanding of exact ethology of the tinnitus also contributes toward this lapse, a general importance of the benefits of an accurate diagnosis can make a lot of things very simple for both the parties. In particular, patients can be on the receiving end, if an accurate diagnosis is not made at an early stage of the disease/symptom.

There are many benefits of an early and accurate diagnosis when tinnitus is diagnosed in conjunction with a number of other symptoms. Some of the most common and outright benefits are explained briefly here:

Reversibility

Usually tinnitus and most of the symptoms in relation to it are reversible if detected at an early stage. The circumstances and factors that influence and produce these symptoms, might be completely reversible if treated early, or they take shorter duration of treatment to control the symptoms and improve quality of life. After a certain period of time, a disease can reach a stage where some of the symptoms may persist for months or in the worst cases years.

Treatability

A few causes of tinnitus are irreversible, but they are definitely treatable. A timely treatment is only possible after a timely diagnosis. Initially, it stops symptoms deteriorating, and then symptoms can be alleviated at later stages of treatment.

Effectiveness

It is a widely accepted rule in medical science that an early and accurate treatment usually leads to higher success rate in treating any disease and the same is true for tinnitus. When effective treatment regimens and medicines are available, the importance of an accurate and early diagnosis increases greatly. Unfortunately, there were not enough effective treatment options available previously. But now things have changed with the launch of newer treatments that are both effective and safe, i.e. 'Natural Quiet'.

Time dependency of accuracy in diagnosis

In the case of tinnitus, it is very rare that the symptom is presented as a single problem faced by a patient. Usually it is accompanied by a number of other symptoms as described in the previous chapters. As the time passes and the disease enters the complication phase, a few more symptoms can further complicate the diagnosis. So it simply means that the earlier a diagnosis is made, the more accurate it will be. Once multiple symptoms develop, accuracy is harder to achieve.

Empowerment

An accurate and early diagnosis enables the patient, himself, to make all the decisions pertaining to his disease; financial, legal and medical/surgical. This empowerment can contribute significantly in long term management planning of the disease.

Resource prioritization and management

Patients can reprioritize their health management options better and at the same time make informed decisions about certain choices that might otherwise be made in ignorance. This also includes choosing and making commitments that can be detrimental to their disease.

Research participation

Those patients who are diagnosed with tinnitus early, can opt to participate in clinical trials aimed at improving treatment options and can take advantage of newer treatments options. A few natural and herbal treatments are proving exceptionally good in tinnitus treatment and management ('Natural Quiet').

Awareness campaigns

These patients can also contribute in spreading the awareness in people about tinnitus and advocate for early diagnosis and its advantages.

Relationship management

Early and accurate diagnosis also prevents extreme stress to build, as family members tend to know more about the disease and treatment options available for the patient. It can help in planning better management of the disease and the patient.

All of the above factors contribute towards better care provision. Together they ensure a better quality of life for the patients.

How to diagnose tinnitus

As we have previously discussed in the earlier chapters, in the majority of the tinnitus patients, the exact cause of the disorder is not known, so when a patient complains of ringing in the ear, he usually goes to an ENT (Ear, Nose and Throat or Otolaryngologist) specialist. Diagnosis begins with a thorough clinical investigation comprising of complete history, physical examination of the ear and use of any medication. A number of tests are available to assist physicians in making an accurate diagnosis. Some of these tests are general in nature, while others are specific to tinnitus:

- audiograms
- evoked response audiometry
- maskability of tinnitus
- residual inhibition
- tinnitus loudness match
- visual analog scale
- tinnitus pitch match
- imaging tests

Audiogram

A hearing acuity test or an audiogram is performed to measure the patients' ability to hear different speech sounds. Sounds are played for one ear at a time and are specific in their nature. If the primary cause of tinnitus is hearing loss, then this test can be very helpful, if not, even then it is performed to rule out certain causes of the disorder.

Evoked response audiometry

This test is performed most of the time for people who have tinnitus in one ear only. It involves computerized inner ear recordings that help the computer to identify any physical abnormality in the particular ear. It resembles fault finding checks performed at garages on cars with computerized engines.

Maskability of tinnitus

This test aims at defining the level at which other external sounds can mask the tinnitus. It is a pain free test that uses a band width of 2000 to 12000 Hz through earphones on the affected ear or ears. The band width is increased gradually to a point where patients can detect the masking sound. Now the pitch of this masking sound is gradually increased until the patient can no longer hear the tinnitus sound. The masking level helps in identifying the severity of tinnitus. "The minimum masking level (MML) is expressed in dB sensation level (SL). In most people, the MML is 8 dB SL or less. It is rare for the MML to go above 22 dB SL."

Residual inhibition

This is performed after the maskability test and it calculates the amount of time that tinnitus takes to come back after the masking sound is eliminated. The masking is performed at a minimal level and 10 dB are added to the minimal masking level for 60 seconds. If for any length of time tinnitus improves, it is recorded. Extensive masking for longer periods of time can provide long periods (hours to days) of relief from tinnitus to some patients.

Tinnitus loudness match

After identification of a sound that most resembles the sound of tinnitus, the loudness of this external sound is adjusted until it matches the loudness of tinnitus.

Visual analog scale

This test is usually performed after the tinnitus loudness match test. It helps to establish the difference between actual loudness of an external sound and tinnitus sound.

Tinnitus pitch match

In this test patients are exposed to a group of selected sounds that are very close to the pitch of their tinnitus sound. High frequency tinnitus can be more debilitating and severe in nature.

"A good way to imagine the value of this test is to consider that the highest tone produced on a grand piano, cycles at slightly over 4,000 Hz. According to recent data, 74 % of people with tinnitus have a 'pitch match' for their tinnitus at 3,500 Hz or higher. Tones in this range typically have an unpleasant, screeching quality."

Imaging tests

These tests are performed to identify or rule out any structural abnormalities in the ear. Depending on the suspected cause of tinnitus, patients may need imaging tests such as X-rays, CT scan and MRI scans.

Factors complicating the diagnosis

The most commonly occurring co-existing conditions that can complicate the diagnosis of tinnitus are:

Anxiety

Depression

Head noise from intracranial aneurysm or glomus tumour

Hypertension

Ménière's disease

Multiple sclerosis

Muscle spasms in middle ear (stapedius muscle and tensor tympani muscle)

Occlusive carotid artery disease

Otosclerosis

Presbycusis (age-related ear or head noise)

TMJ syndrome

Vascular noise from arteriovenous malformation or
   arteriovenous shunt

Differential diagnosis of tinnitus with other co-existing conditions

There are lots of disorders of a diversified nature that can contribute to emergence of tinnitus as a symptom. A mere list of all the possible disorders that can cause tinnitus is enough to understand the dilemma of a physician set to diagnose the tinnitus.

Trauma causes

   Ear drum rupture/tear/laceration, acute
   Head trauma
   Ear trauma
   Post-concussion syndrome
   Labyrinthine concussion

Electromagnetic, physics, trauma, radiation causes

   Blast injury
   Sound, high intensity/noise
   Dysbarism
   Barotitis
   Sound trauma hearing loss
   Deafness, acoustic trauma, chronic

Infectious disorders (specific agent)

Labyrinthitis, viral

Meningitis bacterial

Lassa fever

Herpes Zoster, geniculate ganglion

Infected organs, abscesses

Otitis externa/acute

Labyrinthitis/all

Otitis media, chronic

Osteomyelitis/petrous bone/Petrositis

Otitis media, acute

Acoustic neuritis/neuronitis

Calvarium Osteomyelitis (Citelli)

Neoplastic disorders

Neoplasms/tumours

Acoustic neuroma

Carcinoma, nasopharynx

Cerebellopontine angle tumour

Glomusjugulare tumour

Allergic, collagen, auto-immune disorders

Autoimmune vestibulitis

Cogan's disease/keratitis/acoustic autoimmune

Metabolic, storage disorders

Hypertriglyceridemia

Congenital, developmental disorders

Cerebral AV malformation

Cervico-oculo-acoustic syndrome

Hereditary, familial, genetic disorders

Otosclerosis

Bilateral Acoustic Neurofibromatosis (NF2)

Episodic ataxia/EA-2/Hemiplegic migraine

Usage, degenerative, necrosis, age related Disorders

Presbycusis

Anatomic, foreign body, structural disorders

Temporomandibular subluxation syndrome

Foreign body, ear

TMJ/Cartilage derangement

Impacted cerumen

Temporomandibular joint ankylosis

Labyrinth fistula

Arteriosclerotic, vascular, venous disorders

Carotid artery dissection/aneurysm

Carotid artery-cavernous sinus fistula

Aneurysm, cavernous sinus, int. carotid

Aneurysm, internal carotid artery

Aneurysm, vertebral artery

Carotid artery aneurysm
Internal auditory artery occlusion

Vegetative, autonomic, endocrine disorders

Migraine headaches/syndrome
Labile hypertension syndrome
Hypothyroidism (myxoedema)
Hypertension, malignant
Ménière's disease
Migrainous stroke/ischemic injury
Acoustic migraine
Hypertension, accelerated
Migraine equivalent
Pseudotumorcerebri/Benign Intracranial Hypertension
Vertebrobasilar migraine syndrome
Migraine, hemiplegic type
Migraine, ophthalmoplegic/ophthalmic

Reference to organ systems

Anaemia, severe
Eighth nerve disorder
Pernicious anaemia
TMJ arthritis/synovitis

Eponymic, esoteric disorders

Vogt-Koyanagi-Harada syndrome

Hierarchical major groups

Cochlear disorders

Drugs

Aminoglycoside antibiotic Administration/Toxicity

Aspirin (Acetylsalicylic acid) Administration/Toxicity

Drug reaction/Side effect

Loop-diuretic Administration/Toxicity

Lithium toxicity/overdose

Salicylate intoxication/overdose

Quinine Administration/Toxicity

Salicylate Administration/Toxicity

Quinidine (Quinaglute/Cardioquin) Administration/Toxicity

Poisoning (specific agent)

Monkshood/Aconite herbal/intake

Nicotine/tobacco intake/poisoning

Cinchona/Cinchophen herbal/intake

Carbon monoxide poisoning/exposure

Endrin poisoning

Gila-monster bite/poisoning

Heavy metals ingestion/poisoning

Methyl salicylate ingestion

Organ poisoning (intoxication)

Ototoxic medications/drugs

Drug induced Hearing loss

LIST SOURCES

Google

Wikipedia

Merck

PubMed (National Library of Medicine)

NGC (National Guideline Clearinghouse)

Medscape (eMedicine)

Harrison's Online (access medicine)

NEJM (The New England Journal of Medicine)

Merriam Webster Online Medical Dictionary

The relatively complex processes of auditory completion and hypersensitivity are shown in a relatively simple schematic model (see Figure 1).

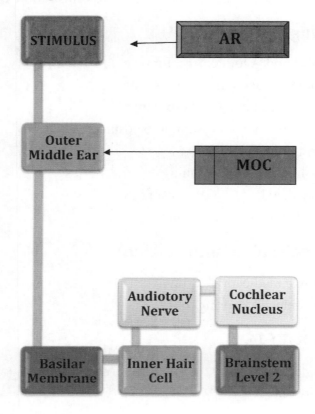

7 Traditional Treatments of Tinnitus

Here is a brief preview of traditional ways that have been used for the prevention and treatment of tinnitus.

Medical treatments

There is no drug-related cure to tinnitus; some drugs can help reduce the severity of tinnitus but will not completely cure the condition. Drugs such as tricyclic anti-depressants, they can alleviate the intensity of tinnitus followed by some side effects like blurry vision, dry mouth and at times cardiac problems.

Alternative treatments

1 Using aspirin to treat blood vessel ailments that can cause tinnitus.

2 Changing medications that may cause tinnitus.

3 Removal of ear wax.

Tinnitus due to medical treatments

Different medical treatments are thought to increase the chances of accidental triggering of tinnitus. Following are some of these treatments:

Ear suctioning

Ear suctioning is a treatment that is recommended to patients who have ear infection problems. It is a safer alternative therapy to syringing and insertion of ear grommets. The noise that is produced at the tip of the suctioning device is loud enough that it can disrupt a patient's ability to hear and 'feel' of ringing sound just as in tinnitus can be felt. If such damage occurs it will be because of the sound energy produced at the suction tip.

Ear syringing

It is not fully proved that syringing can start the onset of a tinnitus condition, but several patients have attributed it as the cause. This type of tinnitus is because of internal physical damage of the ear. An ear syringing procedure can damage the tympanic membrane severely if not carried out by a professional. Tinnitus will carry with it symptoms like vertigo and headache, if it is induced by internal damage by an instrument like the ear syringe.

Grommet insertion

A grommet is a device used to relieve Eustachian tube dysfunction. It is said to reduce any pain associated with tinnitus. Sometimes the insertion of a grommet may become a cause of triggering tinnitus. In this situation the tinnitus will subside if the grommet is taken out carefully and the created hole is covered with rice paper.

Local anaesthetic

An injection of local anaesthetic in the ear canal is very painful if the patient already has tinnitus. The pain can last for several hours and it may also cause vertigo, this will cause lot of agonizing pain for the patient. New topical anaesthetics have lowered the risks built by the local anaesthetics that are inserted directly into the ear canal.

Correcting hearing loss

Correcting of hear loss can be achieved if the right environment is provided to the patient. It can be a gradual training of the patient to acclimatise to newer, better conditions.

De-sensitization of the auditory system

Some patients have a problem with loud high pitched sounds and this averts them from going to public places such as theatres, malls, concerts, public events etc. Therapists must address the patient about their condition that makes them this way. It is the damage to their auditory system more specifically to the outer hair cells. Sometimes people who have this ailment can develop severe phonophobia and may take relief from all social gatherings and from work and often wear ear plugs to keep the disturbing sounds out of their life. To help the patient cope with this condition some recommendations are posed:

- In order to de-sensitize the auditory system it is advised that a patient should listen to pleasant music and sounds such as of waterfalls, raindrops and ocean waves.

- These pleasant sounds can be heard with the help of devices such as sound generators that can be placed under pillows or mattresses during sleep time.

- Patients are motivated to resume social life and again take part in other social activities. It is not a healthy option for a person to be secluded just because of his/her photophobia.

Reduction of noise

For some patients excessive exposure to high frequency of sounds can lead to increased severity of their tinnitus. Clinical experts suggest that such patients wear protective ear plugs and ear muffs to help them avoid the dangers of high pitched sounds like tyre screeching, glass breaking, gunshots, chain saws etc. These loud noises can damage the sensitive ear hair cells that can cause permanent damage to hearing ability.

Sound therapy

Tinnitus sound therapy is usually used to cure this ailment; causes of tinnitus are numerous including loud noises, damage caused by mechanical cleaning of ear and some types of medications.

White noise sound therapy

White noise therapy is used to cure tinnitus with the help of combining different types of frequencies of sound. This mixture of sound helps in hiding or eliminating the ringing and buzzing sound of tinnitus. The tinnitus white sound therapy can be explained to the patient by a professional on how to use it. The white sound therapy is usually available on CDs.

TRT (tinnitus retraining therapy)

TRT works with other modes of therapy; it is used synonymously with counselling and sound therapy. It does not work directly to alleviate tinnitus but it helps the patient to understand the problem and how to deal with it. This therapy educates the patient to stop having negative thoughts about tinnitus because of the fact that the more irritated a person will get, the more severe tinnitus will be encountered.

CBT (cognitive behavioural therapy)

CBT works by helping the clinical expert to determine a patient's condition by analysing the beliefs, thought patterns, and the behaviour one poses in public.

The person's emotions are analysed by therapeutic sessions that can be one-on-one or at group meetings. This kind of therapy is carried out by psychotherapists and clinical psychologists. A modified form of CBT is sometimes also called PTM or Progressive Tinnitus Management, this therapy includes sound as an additional tool to deliver solution. Furthermore there are four types of CBT techniques that are used to treat tinnitus effectively.

Cognitive mind enrichment

This therapy is based on the fact that people have multitude of thought processes going on in their minds. Some positive and some negative; positive thoughts are a healthy sign for a tinnitus patient but negative thoughts give rise to more severe tinnitus. For instance, a person has several thought processes going on in his mind and in the midst of these thoughts a person waking up in the morning would think that today was going to be the worst day of his life - this inner speech refers to self-talk. Self-talk is represented as a negative source of thought. This negative thought stream is linked with self-questioning. A person will question himself whether it is OK to go out today? Or will I come home alive today? These are the type of questions that boggle the mind. Doubt is the outcome of these questions and even though the tinnitus patient may have a mild symptom of the disease he will start to develop the signs of a severe form.

Cognitive mind enrichment therapy is used to address and make believe the people who face this condition that this can be cured. The cure comes in the form of supplementing ones negative thoughts into positive thoughts. The aim of this treatment is not to take the persons mind to a euphoria state but to help him in thinking realistic and positive thoughts or at the most neutral thoughts.

Distraction mind enrichment

Distraction as the word suggests is a tactic to divert attention from one focus to another. Distraction mind enrichment therapy does just that. It is a natural phenomenon when a person concentrates on a certain thing and that thing becomes more and more intense. The same is in the case of tinnitus; the more one focuses on it the more problematic it becomes. Take the example of a person who walks daily from home to work; his body will automatically work on its own even when he is talking on the phone with someone and walking. This mental ability is called a flow state. Being in a flow state you won't remember what was happening around you when walking to work. The therapists exploit this ability of mind and try to train the patient in adopting this method to ward off tinnitus.

The less the mind thinks about tinnitus the less the person will get affected by this havoc.

Counsellors teach tinnitus patients how to think differently; they teach them about the distraction which will make them think of other things other than their condition. People sometimes have their own distraction strategies and methods like counting numbers, going through alphabets, names of animals or flowers etc. Distraction can also include constructive hobbies like gardening, travelling, sports and many other activities.

Relaxation mind enrichment

Nothing seems better than to relax once in a while. A stressed out mind sometimes becomes a source of several ailments of which no cure is available except therapeutic relaxation. It is still an ambiguity whether stress causes severe tinnitus or vice versa. This is more of a chicken and egg riddle of which came first. The point is that they seem to develop together as one, and ways to lessen the intensity are necessary to find.

Counselling specialists can teach how to relax the mind. Various methods are used to address this issue the most common being the progressive muscle relaxation. In this therapy the therapist teaches the person on how to relax different muscle groups in the body. Scanning can be used to detect the stressed parts of the human body and conduct therapy on them for relaxation. Studies suggest the muscle relaxation technique is more helpful when used along with other tools of treatment, like helpful audio/video material, breathing techniques etc. Meditation, yoga and deep breathing have been used by many for body and mind relaxation. A therapy specialist can teach a person how to use these tools properly to mitigate tinnitus. These exercises are done in a noise free environment and it depends from person to person that how the effective they are. Some people may find it boring and more stressful to sit down quietly and think about nothing. For these people casual methods are used, e.g. walking the dog, relaxing in a warm bath, drinking tea, getting cosy in a blanket etc.

Different tools have different effects and these tools are used with combinations that work best for each individual.

Imagination mind enrichment

This method involves making a person imagine good things. The process includes specific imagery and visualizations to soothe and calm the mind. This technique is often used with people who have complains about phobias, stress and depression. The therapist may help a person in creating imaginary mental imagery or visuals that involve all the five senses i.e. touch, taste, smell, sight and hearing. For pleasing thoughts, people might think about things that they enjoy doing like holding their children, patting the dog, going for a walk, and gardening; these are similar to reminiscing moments of joy.

The other end of this method is the negative visuals that you might have during a tinnitus attack. Like writing on a blackboard or screeching of tyres, breaking glass, bees buzzing etc.; here the therapist will help the patients overcome these visuals and replace them with the good ones. This exercise is very helpful in controlling tinnitus if used along with other tools. Tools such as photographs, videos and paintings can help to create a greater positive approach towards the cure.

ATA's Roadmap to a Cure

Roadmap Paths

Roadmap Path Details

Path A
IDENTIFICATION OF TINNITUS GENERATOR(S): Determine sites in the ear or brain where tinnitus-producing signals arise.

A1. Identify areas in the auditory system exhibiting tinnitus-related abnormality.

A2a. Measure the changes in activity identified in A1.

A2b. Use or develop scientific metrics to assess tinnitus percepts in human or animal subjects with abnormalities identified in A1.

A3. Demonstrate that measures of tinnitus established in A2b are causally related to the abnormalities measured in A2a.

Path B
ELUCIDATION OF MECHANISMS OF TINNITUS GENERATION: Determine the nature of abnormal signals and their underlying cellular and molecular causes.

B1. Identify neural or cellular populations giving rise to tinnitus-generating signals.

B2. Determine the altered cellular processes in the cell populations defined in B1.

B3. Define the cellular triggers that induce the alterations identified in B2.

Path C
DEVELOPMENT OF THERAPY: Assess the potential of intervention, manipulation, or treatment as a means of suppressing tinnitus.

C1. Test therapeutic approaches to suppress tinnitus (electric/magnetic stimulation, drugs, surgery, acoustic stimulation).

C2. Use these approaches to target tinnitus generation sites defined in Path A.

C3a. Determine magnitude of therapeutic benefit of tinnitus treatment.

C3b. Assess side effects or risks associated with treatment.

Path D
OPTIMIZATION OF THERAPY: Define parameters of treatment that optimize suppression of tinnitus and minimize side effects.

D1. Refine therapeutic approaches to target specific tinnitus generators identified in Path B.

D2. Improve mode(s) of treatment delivery to reduce any side effects identified in Path C.

D3a. Establish dose/response relationships to maximize benefit and minimize side effects of treatment.

D4. Customize treatment to individual.

8 Natural Remedies of Tinnitus

Researchers have found several ways to manage tinnitus. Tinnitus is a complex condition physiologically and hence there is no single approach. Effective remedies have been sorted out in past years. It is surprising that natural ways have endeavoured far better results than anything else. Moreover, people believe and are accustomed in using natural remedies for treating this condition. That may include diet modification and life style modification also combined with other therapies. ('Natural Quiet')

A Importance of diet for tinnitus patients

Tinnitus is not an illness, but rather a condition that causes a constant noise that only the patient can hear. Scientists have determined that tinnitus is caused by a nervous system disorder involving misinterpreted brain signals between the brain and the nerve cells.

Although there is no cure for tinnitus, health experts have found a connection between certain food ingredients in our diet and tinnitus severity.

Foods to avoid in tinnitus

To reduce tinnitus ear ringing, fullness, or ear pain, try eliminating the following tinnitus diet triggers in food and medicine:

- Salt; especially when hypertensive, is a tinnitus trigger
- Refined white sugar causes blood sugar spikes and promotes Type 2 diabetes.
- Fried food; replace animal fat with vegetable oil such as olive oil, sunflower oil
- Dairy food
- Nicotine is a non-diet tinnitus trigger
- Non-steroidal anti-inflammatory drugs (NSAIDs) especially ibuprofen
- Quinine medication is a known tinnitus trigger
- Caffeinated beverages trigger tinnitus by increasing stress and anxiety
- Alcoholic beverages increase your chances of suffering from tinnitus
- Artificial sweetener should also be avoided

Foods that can improve noise in ears

Start your new diet plan by introducing a high protein diet of beef and beans (e.g. soya beans), broccoli, and other vegetables like spinach, carrots, radish, garlic, potatoes, and eggplants (aubergines).

- Introduce foods high in Vitamin A, Vitamin B12 and Zinc

- Add nuts (walnuts, almonds)
- Fruits rich in vitamins and zinc (such as bananas, figs, apples, plums and raspberries)
- Choose low-fat, low-cholesterol and high-protein meat such as turkey, tuna, salmon, and chicken

Tinnitus supplements

According to naturopathic physician William A. Mitchel Jr., author of "Plant medicine in practice", Gingko biloba is a dietary supplement that has historically been used in treating this condition. Other dietary supplement that may be helpful includes coenzyme Q10, manganese, magnesium, a multivitamin and mineral complex, Echinacea, and Vitamin E. ('Natural Quiet')

Vitamin A

The cochlea in the inner ear stores a large amount of Vitamin A. It relies on sufficient stores in order to receive and interpret sound efficiently. Noise induced trauma is closely related to reduce cochlear blood flow due to excessive noise exposure. Vitamin A in conjunction with Vitamin E is an effective tinnitus treatment and minimises the effects of noise induced hearing loss.

Sources of Vitamin A are spinach, orange fruits, tuna fish and vegetables like yams, carrots and pumpkins.

Vitamin B12

Vitamin B12 is essential for a healthy nervous system. It affects the way we touch, see, taste and hear, so its deficiency leads to irreversible damage to the brain resulting in symptoms such as altered taste, numbness, tingling, visual disturbance and chronic tinnitus. Therefore Vitamin B12 helps chronic tinnitus and noise induced hearing loss effectively in combination with other minerals.

Sources of Vitamin B12 are lean meats, fish, eggs and dairy products.

Magnesium

Nutritionists believe that magnesium deficiency corrupts the ability of the cochlea to function properly by constricting vessels that lead to the inner ear. It helps to minimize the damaging effects caused by noise induced hearing loss.

Sources of Magnesium are brown rice, bananas and oats.

Zinc

Zinc is another nutrient that is required for the functioning of cellular processes, helping the immune system, wound healing and growth. It is also present in auditory paths of brain and the cochlea, so its deficiency is also associated with tinnitus. A featured study showed that low levels of zinc could be the cause of tinnitus. The University of Michigan Health System reported in 1985 that 25% of tinnitus sufferers noticed a marked reduction in tinnitus symptoms when they increased their zinc intake.

Sources in which zinc is highly present are oyster, wheat germ veal liver and sesame seeds.

B Exercise therapy

In numerous ways, physical activities make a visible improvement to worrisome tinnitus. Exercise brings back the balance of the body and relieves stress. Exercising will keep the body active and improves blood flow to the structures of the ear. There are a variety of options, to choose from, i.e. walking, jogging, swimming, martial arts, sky diving, gymnastics, aerobics, dancing, yoga, stretching, fishing, rowing, golf and any sport that helps to stretch your body will keep you active and distract you from the bothersome ear noise. But before adapting anything, make sure it is safe for you and reduces the symptoms, rather than complicating them. Bike riding and sky diving may exaggerate the tinnitus severity as they are noisier activities so be careful and consult your doctor first, before selecting the type of exercise that is best for you. It is important is to select the activity that will help you to relax the most and in the easiest way. Choose only that activity that you really like, so that you can enjoy doing it, and can continue it for longer period of time. Make sure that you get a professional instructor, and proper equipment and clothing so that best results can be achieved. Getting fitter will give you a healthy heart and lungs, better blood flow, and a better stress free personality. It will provide increased muscular strength, flexibility, and tolerance of the body, helping to reducing the severity of Tinnitus.

Following are simple relaxation exercises:

1. Relax in a comfortable position, breathe in slowly; tightly

grasp your hand so that you feel the tension in your hand and wrist then breathe out and relax your hand. Repeat the same with other parts of the body.

2. Breathe slowly, and deeply, and then let it out after holding it for a minute. Wait for a moment and breathe in again slowly and deeply, and so on.

C Herbal remedies

Focusing on other treatment options, herbal supplements are generally effective in improving the symptoms. There are varieties of herbs that are useful in treating tinnitus. To get the best results you should use the herbs that help in improving blood circulation and also provides a nutrient rich diet.

Following are the herbs that could be used to treat tinnitus:

Sesame seeds

Sesame seeds are frequently used by Chinese herbalists, and also in the Indian Ayurvedic system. Sesame seeds are used to treat tinnitus, dizziness and blurred vision. They can be used in food so that it is easier to take. Tahini is the famous peanut butter-like spread that is made from sesame seeds, and Halvah is another popular sesame candy.

Lesser Periwinkle

Lesser Periwinkle (Vinca minor) contains a chemical known as Vincamine. This extract is commonly used by German herbalists to treat Tinnitus and Ménière's Disease. A dose of 20mg of the dried herb is taken three times a day. The side effects of this herb extract include changes in blood counts. There is evidence of a severe decrease in blood pressure, if the extract is taken in high doses, so be careful and consult your doctor - avoid self-medication. If toxicity occurs, then gastric-emptying will be needed.

Other herbs used for treatment of tinnitus include:
- *Gingko biloba*
- *Black cohos*h 3 times a day
- *Golden seal* used in combination with black cohosh (1:1)
- *Sunflower seeds* with brewed tea from their hulls
- *Spinach* and other Zinc containing foods, such as papaya, cucumbers, cowpeas, and asparagus
- *Fenugreek seed tea* 2 times a day
- *Castor oil* 3-4 drops in each ear
- *Onion juice* 1 drop, 3 times a week
- *Passionflower* extract
- *Horsetail* 3-4 capsules daily
- *Ramson juice* 1 tbsp. daily
- *Plantain*
- *Mistletoe tea,* 3 teaspoons mixed with 3 cups of cold water and left over night, then strained the next morning, warm it and drink 3 cups daily.

Herbs to avoid are:
- caffeine
- cinchona

- black haw
- uvaursi

D Homeopathy

Homeopathy works on the principal that the patient is best
treated by the remedy which causes it - 'like cures like'.
Another theory that is the basis of homeopathy is that small
doses of homeopathic medicines are more effective than large
doses of any other medicine – 'less is more'. Although these
remedies are given in high dilutions so they may not contain
any original molecule. Homeopathic doctors believe that your
body has the capacity to cure itself when left alone and
symptoms of a disease are actually signs showing that your
body is attempting to cure the disease itself.

The following are a few of the numerous remedies for tinnitus
according to Dr Barry Rose of the Royal London Homeopathic
Hospital:

- Carbosulphuricum 12c: for buzzing and singing noises
  with defective hearing
- Chininumsulphuricum 12c: for violent buzzing, ringing
  and roaring with defective hearing
- Salicylic acid 12c: for roaring, ringing, deafness and
  dizziness
- Lachesis 12c: for roaring, ringing and excessive ear wax

Take an appropriate remedy twice a day until your symptoms

improve. If there is no improvement then you should consult your homeopath for proper treatment. Other homeopathic medication for tinnitus include; *graphites* for deafness, *coffeacruda* for disturbed sleep with tinnitus, *lycopodium* for roaring tinnitus, and *calcarea carbonic* for cracking noise.

E Acupuncture and acupressure

Acupuncture is an ancient form of healing first used in China more than 2,000 years ago. It works through the insertion of very fine needles into various areas of the body are called **Acupoints**. Acupoints are pressure points in the head, neck and shoulder that are of great importance in reducing mental and physical stress. It works on the rebalance of the forces at work within the system. The important meridians that are related to tinnitus are kidney meridian and liver meridian, their imbalance results in tinnitus symptoms. This therapy is very popular and is done by a licensed acupuncturist. Acupuncturists use different techniques of acupuncture and functions of acupuncture points. For example empty tone; dispersing energy preserve, unblock the meridians circulating blood and energy.

Acupressure is an ancient healing art that is used to stimulate specific key points on the body with the aim of relieving pain and discomfort. Pain and discomfort are the signs of energy imbalance, that if not treated may result in disease or serious illness. Acupressure deals with this energy imbalance by identifying Acupoints. These are located on the channels that run throughout the body and connect all the body parts together. Acupoints are the specific spots on the body that often treat pain or discomfort elsewhere and by addressing the imbalances at acupoints, you can balance the flow of energy and thus reduce pain in an affected area.

Many people confuse acupressure with acupuncture. These two are similar and closely related and both rely on the same fundamental principles as both use the same points and meridians. The main difference between Acupressure and Acupuncture is that Acupuncturist use pins that are hair-thin and sterile needles, whereas an Acupressurist doesn't use pins or needles just pressure points.

This difference is crucial because the needle aspect is something that makes many people nervous about acupuncture. For these people acupressure is an equally effective alternative treatment.

F Reflexology

The majority of physical and emotional tension comes from the stress in our daily life. Stress becomes very harmful if you don't have proper time to relax and recover from stress. Without rest, muscles get weak and become a site for potential injury or damage as muscles need time to rest and repair. Monitoring tinnitus and continuing to worry about it, results in severe tension and stress, and that may make someone physically exerted. To help relieve this tension, you can use simple relaxation exercises to relax. One easy way to reduce the impact of stress is to take acupressure breaks and reflexology, to feel better and relaxed, as stress tends to build up in the muscles of shoulders and neck, causing neck pain and headaches. In alleviating pain and noise of the ear(s), acupressure and reflexology techniques play a very important role. Reflexology began in the United States in the early 1900s.

Reflexology is based on the assumption that organs, glands, and nerves of the body are connected with the reflex areas on the bottom of your feet and palm of your hands. Each of these 'reflex areas' is related to a specific part of the body. Healthy functions of the body can be restored by simply massaging that area. The good thing about the reflexology is that you can perform it yourself and needs no special training or techniques. You just need to know the area affected and where the massage is needed.

The following are the simple steps to reduce the symptoms of tinnitus through foot reflexology:

- Sit in a comfortable position either on chair, sofa or on the floor.
- Cross one leg over the other, resting your foot on the other knee.
- The spot that is said to relieve the symptoms of tinnitus is the spot directly below your two smallest toes.
- Massage this spot for no longer than five minutes, and perform the massage only once on the first day.
- On the second day, massage this area for at least five

minutes; increasing the time slightly. Perform this action twice a day.

- Continue to increase the time slowly every day you perform this massage and ensure that you perform it twice a day.

If you want try hand reflexology as well, follow the same routine; the only difference is that you'll be massaging your little fingers. In the same way, start the massage for five minutes on first day - no more and after that, slowly increase the time of massage and perform it twice a day.

Reflexology results in three amazing things:

- it is relaxing
- it slightly increases blood circulation
- it promotes balance within the body

At the end remember that, reflexology does not cure anything, but it helps to relax body stress but if the complications persist, consult your doctor a.s.a.p.

G Aromatherapy

Aromatherapy means 'treatment using scents'; helping to restore normal functioning of the body through the use of scented 'essential oils'. These oils are extracted from wild or cultivated plants, herbs, fruits or even trees. They are prepared to be used as bath additives, inhalants, or massaging lubricants. The scientific and medical aromatherapy is very effective for relieving stress as essential oils have very interesting properties that act on the central, sympathetic, the parasympathetic, and autonomous nervous systems. These active substances results in very strong anxiolytic and hypnotic effects including calming, sedation and relaxing. Massage your ear with selected oils to relief stress and improve your sleep; essential oils have different components such as aldehydes, ketones, lactones, esters, ethers and depending upon the predominating component of oil, they act differently on the body, but the mechanism of the action of essential oils is not yet understood.

Several pure scents and fragrances are blended together for treating Tinnitus with Aromatherapy. The Illustrated Encyclopedia of Natural Remedies recommends the following essential oils for tinnitus sufferers who have blood circulation problems; rose, lemon, rosemary and cypress. These oils are applied by massaging the head, or as vaporizer in an aromatherapy diffuser. When they are inhaled the smell of the oil is entered through cilia, acting on the brain through stimulation of the olfactory nerves. With time, olfactory neurons become sensitive to the scent, and a less concentrated scent is then required.

Follow the following steps of Aromatherapy for Tinnitus:

1. Place oil in your hand and lie down comfortably. Then massage both of your ears simultaneously.

2. Put a little oil on your fingertip and massage inside and outside rubbing gently to feel your ear.

3. Place your index and middle fingers on the bone of the skull behind the ear lobe; then make small circular movements upwards.

4. Slowly slide the fingers from the centre to the periphery and halfway, change the position of the fingers so that thumb is present inside the index finger. Follow step 3 and 4 at least three times.

5. Touch the lymphatic chains gently on each side of the neck, from the angle mandible to the clavicle.

Recommended essential oils are: chamomile, basil, and tansy.

Advantages of massaging with essential oils include:

- stimulation reflexes
- relaxation
- enjoyment
- elimination of toxins

H Hypnosis

Use of hypnosis in tinnitus is not a new concept; it has been used for more than 30 years. Investigators have concluded that hypnosis is often a potent tool specifically limited to the reduction of tension. The aim of Hypnosis is to induce a deep relaxation state in the patient and to minimize the awareness of Tinnitus. It also maintains normal mental activity so that the patient feels relaxed and can work with more concentration. It is just like not noticing the clock ticking, or the way you breathe or blink in your routine life. You fail to notice them until your attention is drawn towards it. In the same way, Hypnosis and Hypnotherapy creates a deep state of relaxation in which the tinnitus becomes quieter. It helps the body to reduce the tension and anxiety caused by Tinnitus. Self-hypnosis and relaxation techniques are taught to the patient to attain that state of relaxation whenever required. Hypnosis can alter the somatic experience as well to the extent that pain is decreased.

Stages of hypnosis are 1) preparation stage, 2) induction of hypnosis and 3) the later stage of induction called 'deepening procedure'. In the third stage, hypnotists advise certain suggestions and instructions and at the end of hypnosis state is the fourth stage in which the patient is alerted again. In the fifth stage the patient is invited to share how he/she is now feeling.

The process of hypnosis includes following steps that are somehow inter-related with one another such as; pure attention, good imagination power, expectancy, compliance, suggestions and trance experience.

Treatment consists of one hour counselling with the physician with a further four weeks of daily home practice by listening to an audio tape for 15 minutes that was recorded during the first one hour session. Self-hypnosis reduces tinnitus more effectively, as compared to the masking techniques but this technique is less effective for patients with certain kinds of depression

9 Why Natural Quiet?

Basis behind Natural Quiet

Natural Quiet is an outstanding breakthrough in the herbal supplements' industry. It has now become a proven solution and a perfect cure for disturbing and irritating noises in the ear.

1 It diminishes the irritating noises of Tinnitus and makes clear sound hearing possible.

2 Lowers the intensity of chirping and buzzing sounds.

3 Completely mutes hissing sounds generated in the ear.

Ingredients:

- Serving Size: 2 Capsules
- Servings per container: 30
- Propriety blend: 1005mg
- Gingko Biloba 24:6
- Hawthorn leaf and flower
- CoQ 10
- Bayberry Bark
- Burdock Root
- Goldenseal
- L-Theanine
- Myrrh Gum
- Homeopathic Blend: Calcarea Carbonica 8X
- Graphites 8X

- Kali Lodatum 8X
- Lycopodium 8X
- Chinchona Officinalis 4C
- Chininum Sulphuricum 5C
- Kali carbonicum 5C
- Other ingredients: Magnesium Stearate, rice flour, Sorbitol and Gelatine.

Research from Boston Medical School Professors

According to Boston Medical School Professors there are many tiny hairs inside the human ear. The combination of these hair cells is generally known as Stereocilia. Stereocilia helps suppress harmful and extra loud noises. There are some viruses and harsh pollutants in our environment that can damage these hairs just like a bone fracture, snapping them into two or more pieces. In this situation damaged hairs rub against each other and results in the generation of tinnitus sounds. Professors from the *Boston Medical College* have come up with great news – 'Natural Quiet' is a perfect cure for Tinnitus, without prescribing drugs and without any hazards of surgery.

Ringing, buzzing, whistling, hissing, clicking and roaring noises, all gradually fade away with new breakthrough discovery of 'Natural Quiet'.

Now your ears go from noisy to normal in just 5 to 7 days. Actually diminishing all those buzzing, ringing and clicking noises that only you can hear! 'Quiet and Complete Sanity' return in One Week's Time! New Wonder Formula shuts down Ear Noise like Aspirin shuts down a headache.

Reference:

1. *Widely acclaimed by doctors at Harvard and Yale Medical Schools*

2. *Boston Medical School Professors*

Neurotransmitter fluid called gamma amino butyric acid (GABA)

GABA is an amino acid that has an inhibitory effect in the synaptic space between adjacent neurons. Almost 40% of inhibitory activity in the brain is provided by GABA. Clinical studies have proven that GABA supplementation can be very effective for a variety of diseases either as a therapeutic agent or as a supportive therapy. It can improve:

- memory and cognitive functions
- fatigue and tiredness
- anxiety, emotional stress and sleep disturbances

GABA production is not usually the problem as it is synthesised in sufficient quantities in the body, but there are some environmental factors that can lead to its fast depletion in the body and subsequently requires supplementation. A GABA deficiency may result in muscle fatigue, nervousness, tinnitus, anxiety, irritability, depressed mood and sleep difficulty. Being a co-factor in a variety of processes in the body, it is vital to nervous system functioning, neurotransmitter synthesis and communication among body cells.

Supplementing with GABA has shown to increase metabolism, improve cognitive functions and induce a general sense of well-being in clinical studies. It implies that GABA has a high nutrition value and when combined with a balanced diet it can greatly improve neurological and psychological functions.

GABA dosage

GABA is a non-essential amino acid and there is no specific RDA. Adult doses of 250 mg to 1000 mg are shown to be effective in treating a variety of symptoms like mental fatigue, anxiety and stress.

Effectiveness

According to a latest research conducted at Boston Medical School:

"New Wonder Formula Shuts Down Ear Noise Like Aspirin Shuts Down A Headache!

Finally, after years of intensive research, medical school doctors discovered a rare, GABA-stimulating biotical that helps thousands of life-long Tinnitus sufferers can free themselves from constant nerve-jangling ear-noise in a matter of days!

Widely acclaimed by doctors at Harvard and Yale Medical Schools - and reported in the AMA's 'New England Journal of Medicine'. This amazing biotical 'tranquilizes' all intrusive ear noise - puts it into a deep, totally silent sleep - turns it off like hanging up a phone! Frees you from the nightmare of never-ending tinnitus outbreaks **ONCE AND FOR ALL!** No more constant ringing, buzzing, humming, clicking, whistling noises rattling in your head; just the wonderful, glorious feeling of being completely normal again!"

Essential ingredients for Natural Quiet

Natural Quiet is formulated in such a way to provide maximum GABA supplementation in a natural way. That's why it has a number of botanical, herbal and natural ingredients that provide GABA supplementation. A therapeutic concentration is achieved through measured quantities of these ingredients to provide maximum and fast relief for Tinnitus patients.

Gingko biloba

Gingko Biloba is the most commonly used herb to treat the depression and hear loss associated with Ménière's Disease or Tinnitus. It boosts the circulatory system and optimizes the performance level and it has been found, that the extract of 120mg Gingko taken per day, is very useful for tinnitus patients, containing 25% flavones glycosides and 5% terpenes that help to minimize stress. Gingko is a slow working herb that can take many weeks or even many months to relieve the patient. It increases the blood flow which results in the decreased severity of tinnitus as low blood flow is one of the causes of tinnitus. The results are sustainable if the supplementation is continued for longer periods.

Hawthorn leaf and flower

Hawthorn is a tree commonly found in northern Asia, Europe and North America. It produces berries, leaves and flowers, all rich in antioxidants. Traditional herbalists have used it since the dark ages in different herbal medicines. These antioxidants are very well known for improving blood flow and strengthening blood vessels; the qualities that can contribute significantly to treat tinnitus.

A clinical trial aimed at monitoring the effects of Hawthorn extract on blood pressure, found it far superior than a placebo. "Hawthorn may help to manage symptoms and improve physiologic outcomes when used as a supporting treatment for tinnitus." "After 10 weeks, the 19 subjects who took hawthorn extract showed a greater reduction in resting diastolic blood pressure than other study members who didn't take it and hawthorn-taking participants were found to have lower levels of anxiety and stress."

It has also been proven to be an anti-atherosclerotic agent and reduces fats from the blood. Thus it prevents the build-up of fatty deposits in the arteries and particularly lowers cholesterol. It's highly likely for people to self-treat themselves after reading the benefits of hawthorn, but a scientific approach is needed to get the best results from the extract as it needs to be used in conjunction with other ingredients to produce quick results for tinnitus patients.

Co Q10

Coenzyme Q_{10} is a fat-soluble compound primarily synthesised by the body and also consumed in the diet. Coenzyme Q_{10} is required for ATP synthesis at cellular level and functions such as an antioxidant in the body.

The body's internal synthesis and dietary intake appear to provide sufficient Coenzyme Q_{10} to prevent deficiency in healthy people. The oral supplementation of Coenzyme Q_{10} increases plasma, lipoprotein, and blood vessel levels and has resulted in clinical and metabolic improvement in some patients with tinnitus. Although Coenzyme Q_{10} supplementation may be a useful addition to conventional medical therapy for tinnitus, additional research is needed.

Roles for Coenzyme Q_{10} supplementation in neurodegenerative disease, hearing loss and diabetes require further research. Although Coenzyme Q_{10} supplementation is relatively safe, they may decrease the efficacy of Warfarin and presently, it is clear that individuals taking treatment for tinnitus would benefit from Coenzyme Q_{10} supplementation.

Bayberry bark

Bayberry bark is traditionally used to provide nourishment, enhance energy levels, promote sense of well-being and improve cognitive problems like sleep disorders, problems of apprehension and tinnitus. The bark is dull brown with vertical orange cracks, and the younger stems bear sharp thorns. Its leaves are considered to be the most potent source of benefits followed by the bark.

"Some of the constituents included are beta-carotene, catechin, pectin, flavonoids (rutin, vitexin [an active constituent], glycosides, kaempferol, quercetin), flavone derivatives (apigenin, luteolin), essential fatty acids, amino acids, amines (phenyletylamine, tyramine, O-methoxyphenethylamine), tannins (condensed proanthocyanidins), oligomericprocyanidins, saponins, cyanogenetic glycosides, many valuable minerals (calcium, choline, chromium, iron, manganese, zinc, phosphorus, potassium, selenium, silicon and magnesium), vitamins B and C."

The role in alleviating the tinnitus symptom is backed up by research that proves that Bayberry bark reduces cholesterol and regulates blood pressure. Thus blood pressure induced tinnitus responds within days after Bayberry bark supplementation. It also converts low density lipoproteins into high density lipoproteins and thus can be used as an effective treatment for strokes.

Burdock root

Burdock Root is one of the nature's best gifts for blood purification and waste removal from the body. It is said to cleanse and eliminate long term impurities from the blood very rapidly through its action on both the liver and kidneys. Blood overburdened by long term deposition of impurities is a major contributor of tinnitus and Burdock Root can rapidly clear these impurities through its actions on the liver and kidneys.

"As a diaphoretic and diuretic, Burdock Root promotes sweating, that helps to release toxins through the skin and also promotes increased urine, further eliminating toxins via the kidneys and bladder. The increased flow of urine relieves both the kidney and the lymphatic system and has many beneficial effects including relief in tinnitus. It rids the body of excess water weight, relieves swelling around joints and alleviates oedema. This makes it very useful for inflammatory conditions, such as rheumatism, arthritis, gout (by flushing uric acid from the kidneys), scrofula and swellings of the neck and throat."

Goldenseal

The natural antibiotic, Goldenseal has numerous benefits. Traditionally used to treat the symptoms of ear nose and throat infections, it's one of the widely used herbs in cold and influenza worldwide. It has proven efficacy in immune system enhancement, in both clinical trials and laboratory studies. The berberien found in Goldenseal is responsible for increasing blood flow to vital organs. It also stimulates lymphocytes to strengthen immune response against a variety of diseases. Referred to as 'King of Mucous Membranes', Goldenseal has a strong soothing effect on inflamed membranes of the ear in tinnitus patients. By reducing the inflammation in the ear, it reduces the severity and duration of tinnitus episodes.

10 Methods to Prevent Tinnitus from Returning

The first question that emerges in our minds is can I help myself with tinnitus? The answer is simple and obvious: Yes I can! Tinnitus patients are not totally at the mercy of their disorder and they can certainly bring improvements and sustainability for their condition on their own. The most influential part starts with realization that a problem is in existence and must be focused and addressed responsibly. The 2nd main step is adaptation of willingness to seek help from an authentic and professional source. Ideally start with consulting a family physician or somebody who is specialized in ENT or more specifically in treating tinnitus. Of course, consulting a tinnitus specialist will be ideal. The doctor will assess the situation and will start your treatment straightaway or will refer you to a specialist relevant to your condition.

In recent years much has changed in understanding tinnitus. Research and development in various fields regarding tinnitus are necessary to minimize problems that are related to it and in certain areas improvements have produced reasons to believe that successful treatments are now available for tinnitus - at least in some patients. These areas can be specified as psychological therapies, hearing aids and in depth classification of sounds and noise generations. All these options are improving each day to target treatments more specifically for each individual suffering from the tinnitus disorder.

Tip for self-care No 1: Managing tinnitus disorder

In order to recover from tinnitus is a necessity to change lifestyles in every way. Tinnitus is one of those disorders that can cause a huge impact on the patient's psychology which is converted into physical disability later. Anxiety and depression can increase blood pressure as well as depression in the patient. Proper consultation and psychotherapy sessions are very helpful in preventing and affirming mental strength to cope up with ringing and noises in the ears.

Understanding and knowledge of anatomy, genetics and the chemistry of tinnitus has established significantly in past few years due to increased research funding both from pharmaceutical companies and the public sector. A large variety of academic papers and psychological counselling procedures have been produced to effectively provide mental support through therapies and drug manufacturers have formulated several antidepressants and mood stabilizers, with minimal side effects for tinnitus patients with stress and depression.

Tip for self-care No 2: Controlling hypertension and cholesterol levels

Most of the present diseases and disorders are due to self-generated courtesy of bad eating habits and negative daily routines. A very handy and logical tip for the prevention of tinnitus and many other physical disorders is controlling high blood pressure. Taking medical prescriptions regularly and maintaining a daily exercise routine can effectively reduce high and mild blood pressures. One hour walks, gym workouts, physical sports, running and other physical activities can become helpful and in addition, changing eating habits along with the cardiovascular exercises, can certainly eliminate and prevent generation of noises in the ears. Foods that are rich in saturated fats and cholesterol should not be consumed to minimize risk factors of both hypertension and tinnitus respectively. So make conscious and planned efforts towards your physical health.

Tip for self-care No 3: Follow instructions on prescribed medications

Following medical guidance from professionals and making sure that you do not miss any doses of medications are two basic points of self-care. If patients of tinnitus have problems of memory loss or tendency to forget things, it is best to place all medications in a small and clean container. Keep this container in a pocket or close by at all times so they are always available and if taking anti-depressants, ask your doctor about the side effects of the prescribed drugs. Use anti-depressants with minimum adverse effects and follow instructions related to dosages and duration. There are many drugs that are prohibited under specific conditions as with certain anti-depressants and mood stimulators – so watch out for those. Medications are very important for prevention reasons, so if you are not satisfied with the results of any drug immediately contact your doctor to get a replacement.

Tip for self-care No 4: Avoid alcohol and focus on intensive care

The human nervous system is responsible for the functioning of all body activities and maintaining their balance. Tinnitus disorder is a direct consequence of its imbalance under stressful conditions. So do not add further stress to it by using alcohol. Alcohol can accelerate such conditions and can make the situation worse. Alcohol and other recreational drugs also reduce the impact of most of the medications and are not recommended at all.

Keep a journal or note pad to keep a record of your diet routine and medications. This will help you keep up with your treatment.

Tip for self-care No 5: On-going care

Use computers and music devices with great caution as once the tinnitus is triggered you have to be very careful to reduce its impact on your life. If any of your family members is a sufferer of tinnitus make sure you show your empathy and concern. Spend some of your time and energy to explain to them about their condition and treatment of tinnitus. Encourage them and provide full support both morally and through your actions. Watching your loved ones recovering from their illness will give you mental strength as well.

Never allow your tinnitus to impact your daily routine. Do not isolate yourself and try your best to join gatherings and attend social activities as much as you can. Activities and social groups that are related to tinnitus are very significant. Gaining knowledge and understanding of this illness and helping oneself and others, will give you peace of mind. This way you will be able to remain in shape and perform responsibly in your life.

Tip for self-care No 6: '**Flare-up**' care

Be sensible and realistic about your illness and recovery time period as it may take a long time. Extra efforts might be needed to achieve certain points of comfort or gain complete recovery. Read more and more literature and articles related to tinnitus, use herbal remedies like Natural Quiet that has no side effects. To prevent tinnitus from returning even if you are fully recovered or even your situation has improved do not expose yourself to the reasons that caused the tinnitus in the first place. If you are suffering with depressive and mood disorders, do not blame yourself. Nobody can have complete control over their health conditions in certain stages in their life, so just keep calm, remain focused, take prescriptions on time and visit your clinician regularly.

Final Word

This book has covered a wide variety of material relating to Tinnitus and whether you live with Tinnitus yourself or it affects someone you care about, my intention is that the information and guidance in these pages has been useful and improved your knowledge of the condition. After all, knowledge is power, which can equip you with the tools required to reduce the impact of Tinnitus on your everyday life.

Understanding the different types of Tinnitus and the possible causes is the first step to treating the condition. We have explored a number of different treatments from the more traditional to natural remedies and tips of how to help manage the symptoms. It will be a personal choice as to what treatment you chose to follow and it can be a long road to Achieving Natural Quiet, but remember just because you do not obtain initial success, that relief can often be found over time. It can be a matter of trial and error until you find a treatment or method of coping that offers you relief, so don't give up.

I hope reading this book will be the start of your journey towards releasing you from the debilitating symptoms of Tinnitus and Achieving Natural Quiet.

Dr Earl Mindell R.PH., Ph.D